PMS

the complete guide to treatment options

SUZIE HAYMAN

PIATKUS

© 1996 Suzie Hayman

Published in 1996 by Judy Piatkus (Publishers) Limited
5 Windmill Street
London W1P 1HF

The moral right of the author has been asserted
A catalogue record for this book is available from the British Library

ISBN 0–7499–1482–3

Designed by Sue Ryall
Dr Stuart's Botanical Tea reproduced on cover by permission of the
East India Company Tea Ltd and Dr Stuart

Typeset by Wyvern Typesetting Ltd, Bristol
Printed and bound in Great Britain by Mackays of Chatham PLC

Contents

Introduction

Over half the world's population experiences menstruation, and most of them, at some time or other, are likely to experience distressing physical or emotional symptoms directly linked to 'that time of the month'. One of the most common of these, and the most baffling, is premenstrual syndrome (PMS). PMS is the name given to a collection of physical and emotional difficulties that occur between 2 to 14 days before a woman's period begins, and which resolve or disappear a day or so after.

If PMS was a *male* condition, there is little doubt that most of today's medical research would be devoted to exploring and understanding it. According to some studies, 75 per cent of all women suffer PMS to some degree. Researchers Woods, Most and Dery, who looked at the prevalence of menopausal symptoms, found that most women are aware of physical changes in relation to their menstrual cycles and that 10 to 20 per cent report physical or emotional symptoms that are severe to disabling. It may bother them for a few years or months at a particular stage in their lives, or it may be a constant feature of every month. This means that each month around 10 million women in the UK aged between 16 and their early 50s have a week or more of difficulty. They can suffer PMS symptoms that can go from mild discomfort to such intolerable misery that half of the most severe sufferers say they have thought about suicide as one way of escaping their problem.

It has been said that over 150 symptoms may be recognised as suggesting PMS. These range from tension, depression and tiredness, to irritability and food cravings, for sweet or salty foods.

Symptoms suggestive of PMS also include headaches, acne, constipation, abdominal bloating, ankle swelling and breast tenderness. During a bout of severe PMS, women may not only be driven to thoughts of suicide and other forms of self-violence, but may also turn their anger and confusion on the outer world. In a study of women in UK prisons, half were found to have committed their offences in the premenstruum – the three or four days before a period begins, when the symptoms of PMS would be at their peak.

The purpose of this book is to examine PMS, what it is and what you can do about it. The main difficulty in trying to help women with PMS is that, so far, medical science has not been able to give a clear explanation of why it happens and exactly what causes this monthly event in so many women's lives. There is very little agreement as to what exactly constitutes PMS and many doctors cannot even acknowledge the condition exists, let alone offer treatment. Those who do agree there is a syndrome that creates problems may still find the subject confusing and be unable to suggest an effective response. Whether we like it or not, we have to consider the question 'Does PMS exist or is there another explanation for the symptoms many women experience?'

There are many schools of thought about PMS. For every explanation of it there is a suggested cure or treatment. This book aims to examine *all* the explanations and *all* the suggested remedies, and to cover every single aspect of a subject that touches everyone – not just the women who suffer from PMS, but anyone who knows a sufferer, their partners, their families and society.

I hope that men will read this book, too. I know from the many letters I receive as the agony aunt for *Woman's Own* magazine that an enormous number of men sneak a look at what is often considered 'women's' reading. This sometimes may be for a laugh and sometimes out of idle curiosity. But mainly it is out of a genuine desire to understand what is happening to the women who share their lives, at home, at work and in the world at large. I welcome male readers to my column, and not only do I also welcome you here, but there are some chapters that are specifically written with men in mind. Few women live in isolation from men, even when they choose to have their primary relationships with other women. To have men understand the menstrual cycle can only be an improvement, particularly since ignorance breeds fear, distrust and anxiety. Men are often dismissive or flippant about menstruation, but this is actually a defensive reaction to something they find intriguing. Periods are a mystery to many men. When you are excluded from something, left out in the cold, you often pour scorn on the subject and make light of it to devalue the very thing you'd actually like to know more about.

Many women endure monthly misery because of their PMS, and this can affect their relationships, their families and their work. The aim of this book is to explore and understand why it happens, and to suggest specific strategies for improvement for any individual, couple or family suffering from the results of PMS. Understanding a situation is often the first and most important step in doing something about it.

1

Setting the scene

Question: Why do women with PMS have such bad tempers?

Answer: THEY JUST DO, ALL RIGHT??!!!!
We laugh at jokes about PMS in the same way, and for the same reason, that we laugh at jokes about death. It's a coping mechanism, a way of dealing with something that frightens or makes us anxious and confused. We need humour to make the subject less scary and more manageable, because for many women, and their families and friends, the reality is so awful.

> 'When my PMS was at its worst, we never really talked about it. I know that the kids and Bill walked round on eggshells for ten days every month, and there'd be these whispers about 'Mum's PMS' but none of us said much about it'.

The first step to understanding what PMS is, what it does and what you can do about it, is to appreciate how the female body works. We also need to understand how and why our experience of being a woman in this society may

1

also lead to emotional conflicts that can show themselves as physical problems.

WHAT MAKES A WOMAN?

Men and women are very similar in many of the essentials. Both sexes have two arms and legs, and a head complete with a brain. Women can be astronauts, just as men can cook, and both are equally able to be excellent, nurturing parents. But there are differences, even though there may be fewer than you think. The most dramatic, of course, is that women conceive, carry and give birth. The downside of this is that women can have period pains, morning sickness . . . and PMS. The reasons for the physical and emotional discomfort experienced by so many women most, or every, month can best be understood if we first look at the female body and the menstrual cycle.

At conception and until around the eighth week of development, a male and a female embryo will appear identical. Then, the cells that become ovaries, womb, vagina, clitoris and the outer lips of the female genitals in one become the testicles and penis in the other. If you just look at the face or the torso, it's often hard to tell the sex of a baby, toddler or little child. You'd need to see the genitals to be certain which one is a girl and which a boy. Differences are important to us, however, so we tend to dress children and style their hair according to their sex and to treat them, and to expect them to act, according to their gender. 'Sugar and spice and all things nice' are the cues we give our girls, so they grow up expecting to be quiet, biddable and pretty, and to look after other people and do what they are told. 'Slugs and snails and puppy dog tails' tell our boys that they are expected to be rowdy, argumentative, and for their failings to be tolerated and accounted for. Children do behave differently and feel dif-

2

ferently about themselves from a very early age. But the sensations they get from their bodies may not be that different until puberty, which is the branch in the track when men's and women's bodies go off in very separate directions.

PUBERTY AND THE MENSTRUAL CYCLE

We are still not entirely sure what changes in the female body trigger puberty and the menarche – the beginning of periods – but it would seem to have some connection with body weight and the proportion of body fat to weight. This is probably why the average age of menarche in the Western world has been coming down steadily. A century ago it was around 17 and has fallen by 3 or 4 months every 10 years. With better nutrition and health care the current average age of puberty is between 12 and 13. It can start, however, at any time between 8 and 18.

The first sign of puberty is usually a sudden increase in height, closely followed by the development of breasts. Hips and thighs will gain a padding of fat, and the face may become fuller. The skin may become rougher in texture and downy hair will become more noticeable and darker around the genitals, under the arms, and on the arms and legs. Some two years after the 'growth spurt', periods will begin. The age at which you experience puberty tends to run in families, so if your mother was an early or late starter, you are likely to be so too.

From the moment your body begins the changes that culminate in your first period, you will become aware of a cycle that eventually settles into a rhythm of its own. Some elements of change, whether the change from a child's body to an adult's or from one part of your monthly cycle to another, are more obvious than others. For instance, you can't help but notice that a chest that was once flat and smooth now has bumps, and that for some days of each month you bleed. But there is a lot more going on under the surface that influences your body and your feelings, all of which is highly significant. You need to understand both and to make the connection, to get a handle on what PMS is, and what you can do about it. You need first, therefore, to look at the surface.

THE REPRODUCTIVE ORGANS

What do you see, as a woman, when you look at your body? The female genitals, also called the vulva, are soft folds of skin each called labia – the Greek word for 'lips'. The inner pair (the labia minora or small lips) are hairless and shiny. The outer sides of the labia majora (large lips) are usually covered in hair. Labia often look a bit frilly or wrinkled at the edges. The labia can be small and neat or may be long, hanging down quite a way. Just as hands, feet or faces vary in size and shape from person to person, so labia vary in size and appearance in different people.

To the front of the vulva, the labia minora joins and forms a hood, protecting the clitoris. The clitoris is a small nub of flesh that is the most sensitive area in a woman and the main site of sexual pleasure. Behind the clitoris there are two openings. The forward opening is the urethra, through which you pass urine, and the next is the vagina, through which you pass menstrual blood, and which may also be the sex and birth passage. The urethra and vagina are usually hidden by the labia, which touch each other when a woman has her legs together.

This much you can see, although you may need to use a mirror or some yoga-style contortions to do so. Using a mirror or going simply by touch, you can explore your body a bit further. The vagina is a flexible tube which slants into the body, along a line drawn from the vulva towards the small of the back. The vagina is at its narrowest in the first few centimetres of its length. Towards the upper two-thirds, it widens. When you become sexually excited the inner area will 'balloon out'. The lower third is rich in nerve endings, while the area towards the top is far less sensitive. That is why you would feel a tampon as you inserted it but not when it is in place. The vagina only extends some 7 to 10 cm into your body. Most women are able to reach to the vaginal vault, which is the end of the tube, with their index fingers. The vaginal vault is a cul-de-sac or dead end, which is why you can't lose a tampon, or anything else, inside you. The entrance to the womb itself is through a tiny canal called the cervical os. This passes through the cervix or neck of the womb. If you pass a finger into your vagina and feel along the front or anterior wall you will find your cervix jutting out into the vagina some 6 to 8 cm inside. It feels rather like the end of your nose when you touch it with your fingers. You could see your own cervix, using a mirror and a speculum (the plastic device that gently holds the walls of the vagina apart so you can see to the end). To go any further, you need surgery, ultrasound or your imagination.

Inside your body, protected by your pelvic bones, lie your reproductive organs, the parts of your body that are actively involved in the menstrual cycle. At the centre is the uterus or womb. Since the uterus has to be able to stretch to accommodate a full-sized baby and its protective fluid, many people think of it as a large, hollow bag. In fact, it is normally about the size and shape of a pear. Imagine a pear, hanging upside down with the stem end pointing downwards and backwards towards your buttocks, and the rounded end pointing up towards the navel. If you clench your fist, hold it just below your navel and imagine moving your hand backwards into your body, you have the site usually occupied by the uterus. It isn't hanging, high and dry, in an empty space, however. The uterus is

5

squeezed and cushioned by all the other essential organs sheltering in the pelvic cavity. Above and around the uterus lie the coils of your bowel and the final part of your waste or back passage, the rectum. Below it is the sex and birth passage, the vagina. And below the front wall of the uterus lies the bladder and the water passage, the urethra.

The walls of the uterus contain blood and lymph vessels, nerves and muscles. One band of muscles runs up the front of the uterus, over the top and back down to the cervix. These are the muscles that move during menstruation, to push out the blood, fluid and tissue fragments that make up the menstrual flow. They also contract during labour to force the baby out. The same muscles contract during orgasm and play some part in the sensations you feel at that time. Scattered throughout these muscular walls are other tiny muscles. Just before your period, these respond to chemical signals by shutting off small blood vessels that lead to the endometrium or lining of the womb. The endometrium lines the entire uterine or womb cavity. It is a soft, pink layer of tissue that is rich in blood vessels. When these muscles cut off the supply of blood, the endometrium begins to decay and come away as the menstrual flow. At the end of your period, further signals cause these muscles to contract even more, stopping the bleeding.

At the top end of its upside-down pear shape, the cavity of the uterus widens out and opens into the two fallopian tubes. These are around 10 to 16 cm long and curve forwards in your pelvic cavity. Each tube is a narrow, muscular channel, and is lined with minute, hair-like filaments called cilia. These move all the time, like the arms of a sea anemone. The movement sets up currents in the fluids moving around in the pelvis, so fluid is pulled down the fallopian tubes and into the uterus. Each fallopian tube ends in finger-like projections called fimbria and close to these hang the ovaries. The ovaries themselves are the size and shape of unshelled almonds – around 2 cm wide and

3.5 cm long. We often refer to the ovaries as 'egg cases', but they do not really contain eggs as such. What each ovary contains is thousands of immature cells that *could* grow into an ovum or egg, given the correct stimulus. Ovaries have in them literally millions of such potential cells at birth and, by the time puberty arrives, some 200,000 still remain. During the average lifetime of a modern woman some 400 of these cells are likely to develop into ova.

The uterus is held in place by the cervix and by ligaments or bands of strong tissue. These are slung across the pelvic cavity from the pelvic walls, the bladder and the rectum. The uterus, the fallopian tubes and the ovaries are all attached to these ligaments. However, none of the pelvic organs are, or should be, stuck firmly in one place. The uterus shifts around, pivoting around the cervix. When you stand up, the uterus will be almost horizontal as long as your bladder is empty. If your bladder is full, it will push the uterus upwards and backwards. A full rectum will squash it down and forwards.

The uterus will also settle under the force of gravity, so if you lie on your side, back or stomach (or stand on your head!) it will press down in that direction. As you breathe, the uterus is pulled up and down in time and, when you become sexually excited, the ligaments tighten to pull the uterus up out of the way of the thrusting penis. The hollow parts or cavities of the vagina and uterus, although normally squashed flat by their muscular walls and the surrounding organs, can at times have air pushed into them. You may notice that lovemaking, especially in some positions, will produce embarrassing sounds as if wind is being passed. If you do a head or shoulder stand while doing keep-fit, especially during your period, the same effect can result. There is nothing worrying or abnormal in this, although it can be extremely dangerous to actually blow air into the vagina.

THE MENSTRUAL CYCLE AND
HOW IT WORKS

'I have always had problems with my periods. When they first started I was always getting period pains and feeling pretty awful. When I had my daughter it seemed to change. I found instead of getting pain when I was bleeding I was feeling awful in the week or so before.'

But if the outer and inner organs are the nuts and bolts of this machine, your body, what about the invisible fuel that sets it ticking? Hormones play a major part in every woman's menstrual cycle. Hormones are substances produced by glands in the body, and they act as chemical messengers, stimulating changes or affecting various parts of the system.

The menstrual cycle starts in a part of the fore-brain called the hypothalamus. The hypothalamus regulates and controls a small gland called the pituitary. This is located in the base of the brain. The hypothalamus produces 'hormone releasing agents' which are chemicals that stimulate the pituitary into producing its own hormones in turn. At puberty, the pituitary begins to manufacture and release into the bloodstream a variety of these chemical messengers – hormones. The hormones' first job is to trigger the gradual change from a child's body to that of a mature woman. One of these changes will be the establishing of regular monthly bleeds and of ovulation – the production every month of a potentially fertile egg. Once started, this gland then controls and regulates periods each month.

It is worth noting that the hypothalamus has a complex 'feedback' relationship between mind and body. It can be affected by both a woman's emotions and her physical state. If either is under stress, the hypothalamus may react by reducing the production of releasing agents, and this has the effect of shutting down or disrupting her whole hormone system. Periods may stop, become irregular, or increase in flow or occurrence, and the woman may find it difficult to start or sustain a pregnancy.

Each menstrual cycle can be imagined as lasting 28 days – day 1 being the first day of bleeding, and day 28 being the day before the next period. In practice, menstrual cycles can vary from 21 to 35 days, although the average is 25 to 30 days.

Menstrual phase

Day 1 to day 5 of the cycle are called the menstrual phase. Stimulated by the hypothalamus, the pituitary produces a hormone called follicle stimulating hormone (FSH). This acts on the ovaries and triggers tiny sacs, called Graafian follicles, which each contain an immature ovum, into ripening. Some 10 to 20 of these may begin to mature. As they do, cells lining the follicles produce another hormone, oestrogen.

Follicular phase

The next phase, which lasts from days 6 to 12, is called the follicular phase. Oestrogen levels rise and the hormone is carried in the bloodstream, and, in turn, acts on the endometrium or lining of the womb. The cells that make up the endometrium respond to oestrogen by thickening and multiplying. After six to eight days, the pituitary stops producing FSH and starts giving out another hormone – luteinising hormone (LH).

Ovulatory phase

This triggers the ovulatory phase which lasts from day 13 to day 15 and causes one of the several maturing follicles on the ovary's surface to burst. This is ovulation, when an egg or ovum is released, and it happens some 12 to 16 days before a menstrual period, and is a woman's most fertile time. Each ovary tends to take it in turn to produce an ovum and only one will mature each month. The ovum will be catapulted into the fluid that circulates throughout the pelvic cavity.

At the time of ovulation, the open ends of the fallopian tubes will have moved closer to the ovaries, and be hovering over them ready to catch the released ovum. The cilia that line the fallopian tubes draw the fluid from the pelvic cavity into the tubes. This wafts the newly released egg down one of the tubes and into the uterus.

Luteal phase

Meanwhile, the luteal phase, which lasts from day 16 to day 23, will have begun. Where the ovum burst out of the ovary there is now an area called the corpus luteum ('yellow body', after its colour). The corpus luteum, the site of the ruptured follicle, begins to manufacture its own hormone, progesterone. Progesterone acts on the ovaries, preventing any more follicles from maturing and ripening. It also has the effect of enriching and priming the lining of the womb, the endometrium, to make it thicker and ready to receive a fertilised egg.

The ovum takes seven to eight days to travel down the fallopian tube from the ovary to the uterus. If conception is to take place, the egg must meet sufficient vigorous and live sperm in the 12 to 24 hours after ovulation. After that, it begins to decay. The egg is at its best in the first 12 hours after ovulation, although it can survive for up to 24 hours. If it is to be fertilised, it needs to meet lively sperm almost as soon as it enters the fallopian tube. If this meeting doesn't happen at the right time in the journey from ovary to womb, the egg will not be fertilised. It will then be washed out of the body in the normal flow of fluid. If sperm is waiting in the tube or arrives soon after, it will surround the egg and one sperm will break through the egg's covering. This is fertilisation. The male cell and the female cell will combine, and the resultant bundle of cells, called a blastocyst, will continue down to the womb.

If the egg *is* fertilised the resulting blastocyst will secrete yet another hormone into the bloodstream. This is called human chorionic gonadatrophin (HCG). HCG stimulates the corpus luteum to continue producing progesterone, encouraging the lining of the womb to enrich itself even more.

Premenstrual phase

If the egg is not fertilised, the corpus luteum shrinks and stops producing progesterone. Day 24 to day 28 is the premenstrual phase, which begins with levels of oestrogen and progesterone falling sharply. When progesterone levels have dropped, tiny muscles inside the walls of the uterus close up and cut off the blood supply to the endometrium. The lining of the womb then falls away as a period – a flow of blood, tissue and fluid. As this happens, FSH levels start to pick up again and the whole cycle repeats itself.

The uterus itself reacts to changes in hormonal levels by flexing and contracting, forcing out the contents of the womb. The shedding process can take between two to eight days, and the amount of fluid and tissue lost may vary from individual to individual, and from period to period, but is usually around a quarter to three-quarters of a tea cup. The womb does not 'store up' blood. If your period is a little heavier than usual one month, it will be because the lining has grown thicker for that month, not because blood has been blocked or held back inside you. A light period is a result of the lining having been thinner in that month.

'When I start bleeding it's like a dam has burst. In the week before my period I can feel myself filling up. It's like my body gets bloated, and I feel sick and heavy and tired. I get tension headaches and I really do feel as if my skin is stretching fit to burst. When the bleeding starts it's like sticking a fork into a sausage. I really feel as if I've been holding my breath and I can let it out. Blood comes out and at the same time all that tension just floods away. My headache goes and my waistbands stop feeling tight, and I can go back to wearing my jeans or a skirt instead of leggings, which are all I can get on in that week.'

The menstrual cycle is a finely balanced, circular sequence. Each stage has a precise function and is caused by natural, normal changes in your body, which you cannot help but notice and come to expect each month. Why, then, should some of us regularly find these changes are accompanied by unpleasant, uncomfortable symptoms? If we are going to understand PMS, and be able to do something about it, there are two questions that have to be asked. First, there is the obvious one of 'What causes it?' Second, there is the more contentious one of 'Does PMS really exist?' Before looking at them, however, Chapter 2 looks at how women experience PMS.

2

Symptoms of PMS

Premenstrual syndrome is not a specific condition or illness, such as influenza or measles. It is exactly what the words mean; a collection of symptoms that come together just before menstruation. There is nothing abnormal about the premenstruum (the five days before your period) itself or about being premenstrual (being at that stage of the cycle). What PMS signifies is an experience of this stage that is uncomfortable or unacceptable.

WHAT ARE THE COMMON SYMPTOMS?

There are said to be around 150 symptoms identified as suggestive of PMS. The list of symptoms started with an assessment form created by Moos, who developed a menstrual distress questionnaire (MDQ) in 1968. The MDQ is a list of 47 symptoms, the result of asking women open-ended questions on the changes they experienced in their menstrual cycle. Seven main factors were identified; pain, concentration, behavioural change, water retention, negative affect, arousal and control. Following on that, Halbreich and his colleagues developed the premenstrual assessment form (PAF). This differs from the MDQ because it defines the timing of symptoms, tying them into the pre-menstruum and making the PAF a tool with which to assess PMS. The PAF consists of 95 items, and according to Halbreich is a reliable and valid way of finding out if PMS is present. Since some of the subsets in the PAF could be divided, for instance you can count nausea and vomiting as one feature or divide it into two, this is why an overall figure of 150 different symptoms now tends to be suggested. These symptoms can be divided into the emotional and the physical.

Emotional symptoms

The most common emotional symptoms reported are as follows.

Depression

'I'm prone to really black moods, feeling really down two to three days every month. It can be quite frightening really and it has very little to do with what's actually happening to me. I had one of these depressions last year when we were on holiday with friends, and I nearly ruined the whole holiday for everyone. As soon as my period started, of course, I felt back to normal. My friends simply couldn't believe that the way I'd been was just the result of PMS.'

Anxiety

'I get panic attacks. I'll be driving in the car or just doing something like the washing up with no reason at all to feel jumpy, and I'll get this wave of terror that goes through me. I start shaking and get butterflies in the stomach, and I can get sweaty and can't breathe properly. I'm not a nervous person, it only happens just before my period.'

Irritability

'I've got a pretty even disposition and I can always tell when my period is due because I get irritable. It's as if I'm grumbling two or three days non-stop and anything my family or friends or colleagues will say makes me snarl.'

Lack of concentration

'My husband says that he knows I'm having PMS when I get hold of the remote control and start zapping. It only lasts a day or so but once a month I just can't settle. It drives him crazy and it doesn't do me much good because I can't keep my mind on anything.'

Memory loss

'Three weeks out of every four I can go round the super-market and get everything I need without having to write it all down. It's just unbelievable how much difference it makes when I'm having PMS. I'll forget the sim-plest things like if one of my flatmates asks me to make a cup of coffee and by the time I've put the kettle on I'll have forgotten why I'm doing it. Or I'll go upstairs to run a bath and end up sorting out my tights.'

Moodiness

'I'm up and down for about four or five days. One minute I can be laughing like a maniac, the next I'm in tears and then ten minutes later I'm screaming at the kids. The funny thing is that I think it would be easier if I was all one thing or the other. If I was angry all the time or down in the dumps all the time at least I'd know where I was and so would they. What makes it so hard is that I just don't know from one minute to the next how I'll be feeling.'

Tension

'Every other month or so I feel like I'm on a knife edge. It's as if I'm really strung up tight and I walk around with my teeth gritted and my hands gripped. The back of my neck gets all knotted up; I can actually feel it.'

Apathy – a 'don't care' attitude

'My mother and I used to have flaming rows about my keeping my room tidy. She always used to say she couldn't understand what got into me because half the time I'd be OK and then I'd be a real slob. It took my husband to point out to me that I'm a real scrub-everything-that-doesn't-move type of person except when my period's due. Then I go into a total slump. I'll lie around watching television, I won't bother to do my hair or face, I'll wear the same sweatshirt and leggings for days, and let everything go. It's no good pointing out to me what I'm doing wrong, because I simply couldn't give a damn. Until my period comes, of course, and then I'm dashing around putting it all right.'

A feeling of being 'got at'

'I go through stages when I think everyone is whispering behind my back and people are picking on me. I'm only like this once a month, thank goodness. Other times I get on well with everyone and they are not a problem.'

Difficulty in making decisions

'I usually have no problem knowing my own mind, but it all goes to pot one week a month. I'll stand in the supermarket, trying to make up my mind whether we're having chicken or chops that night and it's like it's a major decision.'

Negativeness

'It doesn't matter what anyone wants to do, I'll come up with the opposite. I can't help it. I just get in a "no" frame of mind and nothing you do is going to please me. I see the downside of everything and nothing is right. My partner knows better than to try any DIY or start anything in the garden when my period is due because I'll be standing there telling him it's all going to go wrong, it's not going to work, what's the point, it's all useless.'

Anger at others or at self

'You fly off the handle at a moment's notice, that's what PMS does to me. You get in a rage with yourself as well. You stand in front of the mirror just hating what you look like, and you even stamp round the house shouting what a fat pig you are and how disgusting you are. When I was a lot younger I even cut myself once because I got so angry, and I'll hit the children which I'll never do at any other time in the month.'

Violent behaviour

'I got a reputation at school for being a cat because I'd really fly at people and hit and scratch when we had a fight. I was up in court and had to leave my first job because I hit someone I had an argument with. I used to regularly hit my husband, and he'd have cuts and bruises and he'd tell people he'd had a fight in the pub because neither of us wanted to say it was me. We were both ashamed. Then I hit my little girl. I was so frightened I talked to the health visitor. She got the doctor in. I was so scared I thought they'd take my little girl away or lock me up. But he said it was PMS and I just needed help for that.'

Tearfulness

'I'll always cry at sad films, but for three or four days before my period starts I'll cry at anything – and I mean anything. Ads on TV can get me bawling and if my husband has anything to say that's out of place or the kids act up, it just sets me off. It's not something I can do anything about.'

Loss of confidence

'I'm a confident sort of person. You know what you're good at, and in my job you have to stand up in front of people and look like you know what you're doing. Usually that suits me fine. A day or so every month that just goes straight out the window. It starts with me feeling a bit low and not quite as bouncy as usual. So I suppose I'm not on top form for about a week, but on the worst days I simply can't do my job properly. It started last year after I had a baby and it's actually getting worse because I'm getting myself wound up knowing it's going to happen, knowing I'm just not going to be able to do it.'

Lack of sexual feeling

'We used to have a good sex life but what with one thing and another it's gone really downhill. I just don't feel like it. I really don't feel like it for about ten days or so in every month, when my period's due and in the week or so before that. It's not that I don't love my partner, it's just that sex has no interest for me at all.'

Physical symptoms

The common physical symptoms may be as follows.

Headaches and migraine

'I suppose everyone gets headaches at some time or another but I don't really except before my period. I started getting headaches a few years ago and I'd feel bad for a day or so. When I mentioned it to a friend she said she got PMS and she'd have a headache every month just like clockwork. That's when I realised the headaches I was getting were the same. They'd come the day or so before I had a period and the day after I started bleeding they'd just go away.'

Bloatedness

'I blow up like a balloon. I'm so bad that I have two sets of clothes – my PMS clothes and my ordinary clothes. I'm usually a size 12 but I've got sizes 14 and 16 in my wardrobe because otherwise I wouldn't be able to do the waistbands up. I'll gain a few pounds every month and then as soon as my period comes it just goes away, but I'll put on a lot more in size than you'd think from what the scales say. In fact, I've taken my wedding and engagement rings off and forgotten to put them back on immediately, and then found I couldn't get them on until my period comes along. That's how much it makes my fingers swell. When they are on, I wouldn't be able to get them off during that week.'

Breast tenderness

'My breasts don't actually get any bigger, but they feel really sore and I can feel every touch on them, I'm that tender. I usually like it when my husband strokes my breasts when we make love, but if he touches me there just before my period I just hit the roof. It sets my teeth on edge and, to be truthful, it can really hurt.'

Acne

'Lots of people go through this really really spotty stage when you're a teenager and you think you'll grow out of it. But I get spots every month. They are usually on my face, but sometimes I get them on my shoulders or back. They last into my period and usually clear up at the same time as my period's tailing off. And since my period is usually four or five days long I suppose I have them for about a week.'

Bowel problems

'I hate it when my period's due because I get tummy problems. Most of the time I get diarrhoea, although sometimes I'm constipated. It doesn't matter what I eat and it doesn't seem to matter what I do. It goes on through my period and when that stops I go back to normal again. Until the following month, of course, when it starts all over again.'

The frequent need to pass water

'I've had cystitis a couple of times and it's a little bit like that. I just keep wanting to go, but it's not as if I'm full every time. I'll probably go about twice as often as I normally do – maybe more. I find I'll be up in the night once or maybe twice.'

Hot flushes

'I thought I was having an early menopause because I started getting these hot flushes. It's really strange. I'd be sitting doing nothing special and all of a sudden it's like I've stepped into a sauna or something. You can feel your whole body going red and you get very sweaty. I saw my doctor, but since my periods haven't changed and are still regular we worked out that it only happens in the week before my periods. So it's not the menopause, it's PMS.'

Nausea

'I'll suddenly feel sick and once or twice I've even retched a bit. I've never actually been sick but a few times I've thought I would. It happens about one month in three, and it will come back on and off for three or four days.'

Aches and pains

'I get backache quite a lot, not just in the week before my period but also through the month. But it does come more often then. I get odd aches in my knees and wrists as well, and that only happens before a period. Sometimes I feel as if I'm getting flu because it's the same sort of aching feeling, but if it happens a week or so before my period I'm pretty sure it will go away when my period does start, and that's what it always is.'

Increased appetite

'I get the munchies for a week or so every month. I just feel really hungry and I'm always nibbling on something, whatever comes to hand. I'll go through packets of biscuits and if I'm sitting watching television I'll want a slice of cake or some toast even though we might have had a really big meal an hour before.'

Food cravings

'I get these real longings for things. Sometimes it's pasta and the family get fed up because we have spaghetti every night for a week. Or I buy a big bag of crisps for the whole family and eat the lot myself. My friend gets into chocolate. She and her husband came over one night and she brought one of those really big two-pound bars. I think I had about the same as a small bar and my husband and hers each had a little bit more, which left her with about a pound and a half and she ate the lot. I don't think the men could believe it, but I could. She said she'd been thinking about chocolate all day and I knew just how she felt.'

Weight gain

'My weight goes up and down like a yo-yo every month. I can put on half a stone in weight and then lose it all without having to do a thing when my period comes. It drives you crazy because it doesn't matter if you diet or count calories or what. It happens every month and it makes getting clothes really difficult.'

Clumsiness

'My partner always says we have a smashing time when my period is on its way. I don't think a month goes by without me breaking something. I drop things, knock things over, trip over things – you name it. I've trodden on the cat before now. I broke my leg once and I smashed the car up and dropped a really beautiful wine glass that my aunt gave me as part of a set as a wedding present. Every single time my period was just around the corner.'

Tiredness

'I could sleep for the whole week before I have a period. I just feel tired all the time. I feel really wrung out even though I might have done nothing, and then the week after I could have all sorts of things on the go and be full of beans. So I don't think it's me, I think it's definitely PMS.'

Sleep disturbances

'I don't like taking sleeping tablets, but sometimes I think I should. It's only for five or six days, but when I have PMS I really can't sleep. It's like insomnia. I'll go to bed and even if I close my eyes I won't drop off. So I'll try reading or watching television, and then I'll find it's three in the morning and I'll still be awake. At other times in the month I'm fine. I've got a friend who is just the opposite. She is usually up bright and early but she can always tell when her period's due because she sleeps right through her alarm and just can't wake up.'

Many women experience these symptoms, either physical or emotional, separately or in various combinations. They may vary from month to month. Your individual pattern of how PMS may be affecting you will emerge clearly if you start keeping a menstrual diary in the way explained in Chapter 6.

With a list of symptoms as long as this is, there is a danger of falling into the 'medical encyclopedia syndrome', where you read any book about illnesses and within three pages you are bound to be convinced you have anything from acidosis through to Zollinger Ellison syndrome! However, there can be little doubt that a considerable number of women experience these distressing symptoms, both emotional and physical, at some time in their lives. But how can you be sure they are not just part of being a woman or something anyone may experience – an unpleasant side-effect of life itself?

What makes it PMS is if these particular experiences arise from and can be tied into a specific regular occurrence – the menstrual cycle. There may be over 150 symptoms recognised as leading to a diagnosis of PMS, but any and all of them can just as readily be symptoms of anything from flu to stress. The only workable definition of PMS is not the symptoms themselves but their timing. If changes take place and can be seen to occur on a regular basis in the premenstruum (that is, in the days before a period begins), and to improve and then disappear in the days after a period begins, then it can be said that PMS is present.

WHAT IS PMS?

PMS remains a controversial subject among doctors. Dr Katharina Dalton was the doctor who first put the concept of premenstrual syndrome on the map. Her definition is that 'Premenstrual syndrome is the recurrence of symptoms in the premenstruum with absence of symptoms in the postmenstruum'. By her definition, therefore, what symptoms you suffer and how badly you have them is less important than when they happen. For you to be suffering from PMS your symptoms must occur in the four days before your period and be relieved by your period beginning. She also says that for it to be PMS you should be free of your symptoms for at least seven days of every cycle.

There is a problem with this. Keeping strictly to her definition, if you have symptoms beginning *five* or more days before your period and if they continue after, or if any of your symptoms occur haphazardly through the cycle, you don't belong to the club. That's a pretty strict definition because if one of your symptoms is headache you may find yourself being told you can't be suffering from PMS if you have headaches at any other time. This may be a convenient way of keeping the figures tidy, but it doesn't help you.

Another definition of PMS is that it is 'The cyclical recurrence, in the luteal phase of the menstrual cycle, of any combination of distressing physical, psychological and/or behavioural changes of sufficient severity to result in deterioration of interpersonal relationships and/or interference with normal activities'. This is both a broader and a narrower definition. It's broader because the luteal phase of the cycle means any time after ovulation and before the end of a period, and this definition doesn't specify exactly when symptoms begin or end within this time scale. It's narrower because it speaks in terms of 'severity' and that can be quite difficult to judge or quantify.

In yet another definition, PMS is called primary recurrent premenstrual tension disorder and is assessed to be present if:

1 at least five of a possible eight sets of mood and behavioural symptoms are met;

2 overall disturbance is so severe that the woman suffers serious impairment with family, at home, at school or at work and/or seeks or is referred for help or takes medication;

3 has symptoms for at least six out of nine menstrual cycles;

4 suffers symptoms only during the premenstrual period with relief of these soon after the onset of menstrual bleeding.

This particular definition concentrates on emotional changes such as depression and stress. Women whose primary symptoms are physical, such as breast tenderness, aren't counted.

There are plenty of other studies and quite a few other attempts at definition, often with complex names to describe the particular phenomenon we are calling PMS. In *The Diagnostic and Statistical Manual of Mental Disorders*, which is the definitive American guide for doctors on mental and emotional illness, the term Late Luteal Phase Dysphoric Disorder has been introduced. To make this diagnosis at least five of ten symptoms should be present 'for most of the time during each symptomatic late luteal phase'. To make the diagnosis these symptoms should also be present:

1 in most menstrual cycles during the past year;

2 stop within a few days after bleeding begins;

3 seriously interfere with work, social activities or relationships;

4 not merely be symptoms of depression or any other personality disorder.

The problem with all of this is that if you keep changing the definition you can never be sure exactly what you are talking about. The point about a clinical definition is that it doesn't just describe *what* is happening but *why* it happens. The importance of this is that if we can agree on what is happening and why it is happening we may be a good step nearer working out what can be done about it. This, of course, is the problem with PMS. Doctors simply can't all agree on what is happening or why, and therefore, no one can come up with a foolproof cure that works for everyone.

As far as any PMS sufferer is concerned, PMS may have one of several definitions. It can be seen as:

one or several symptoms that begin four days before your period begins and clear up two days after.

Or, PMS may be:

one or several symptoms that begin in the week or so before your period begins and clear up soon after your period starts.

Or, PMS may be:

> one or several symptoms that occur around your period and cause you great distress.

It's fairly obvious that most of us see PMS as a disorder linked to the menstrual cycle. Most doctors refine this definition further. It's not the bleeding that we should be looking at but what is happening in the ovaries. Most of us obviously judge our menstrual cycle by the bleeding because that, after all, may be the only event in the cycle that we can see or feel. The medical profession, however, looks at the wider picture and, if we are to have some understanding of what PMS might be, we need to do this too. PMS, according to many doctors, therefore, is a disorder of the *ovarian* cycle; it is what is happening in the ovaries that is really important.

We seem to know so much about the body that it may come as a surprise to realise that the full story of what happens and why is not completely understood. Simply told, we know that women produce an ova or egg every month and that if this is not fertilised we bleed as the reproductive cycle begins again. We know that hormones or chemical messengers set off and maintain this cycle. We know which hormones do what at particular points in the cycle. But the further we go into the *exact* ways and means, on a microscopic level, the fuzzier the picture becomes.

We have looked at the symptoms; Chapter 3 goes on to consider some of the theories of how and why these occur.

3

Causes of PMS

Every woman will go through a premenstrual phase each cycle she is not pregnant. What, then, makes this experience trouble-free for some women, or for some months; what makes it unpleasant enough to be called PMS in other women, or in some cycles? The answer is that we don't really *know*. There is as much argument over what causes PMS, as what it is and what might cure it.

When trying to understand PMS, its possible causes and treatments, you have to recognise one very important fact. This is that while we may be able to document the obvious 'hard' structure of the body by producing accurate diagrams, and explanations of the skeleton, muscles, tendons and arteries, we do not know the full workings of the biochemistry of the human body. It may be as easy as doing a jigsaw to see how bones and ligaments fit together, but when it comes to comprehending the way hormones affect mood and effect physical reaction, we are still largely learning. This is why, when we talk about PMS, you will find any honest and responsible text peppered with phrases such as 'it is suggested/postulated/theorised/ said'.

Many theories are only theories and have not been, and

cannot with our current knowledge yet be, fully proved or disproved. Many theories are constructed from assumptions and sheer hunch. For instance, investigators might suggest that PMS is caused by the lack of some body chemical, because any symptoms mimic those of a deficiency or a withdrawal of that chemical. Having had that idea, they may look for proof by trying to see if PMS sufferers do have a deficiency, and if giving supplements of whatever it is produces a helpful result. But this doesn't mean that anyone has proved or knows that the chemical is at fault. It's often simply a case of 'Let's see if this works'.

Here are some of the theories.

PROGESTERONE AND OESTROGEN

An American doctor called Israel first suggested that PMS occurs when you have an imbalance in levels of oestrogen and progesterone, with high oestrogen and relatively low progesterone. Quite a few studies have followed this up, and seem to agree that premenstrual anxiety, irritability, depression and bloatedness could be associated with high oestrogen and low progesterone states. However, no other hormones in the body show such variation in levels as these two. Because they go through such a rise and fall, and these changes often parallel the onset and relief of PMS, it's not surprising that oestrogen and progesterone are naturally seen as the culprits. The argument is that when you have a relative drop in progesterone compared to oestrogen, or when for some reason the body is unable to make use of the progesterone circulating in your system, you will get the uncomfortable reactions we know as PMS. However, the evidence is inconsistent and is still inconclusive.

Women may start to experience PMS, or may find their PMS worsens, after a pregnancy and one explanation for this has to do with the way that the body uses progesterone. Hormones, such as progesterone and oestrogen, are chemical messengers, which means that they carry an instruction which is received or taken up by particular cells. These cells are called receptors.

When you get pregnant the level of progesterone in your body increases enormously, as messages to establish and then maintain a pregnancy are carried and received. The theory is that receptors get flooded with so much progesterone that they build up a tolerance. This means that in future they may need more of the hormone to have the same effect. When, after the pregnancy, you go back to a usual level, it's not enough and your body acts as if there is an imbalance or a deficiency in progesterone.

PROLACTIN

Another explanation for PMS is that it is caused by high levels of the hormone prolactin. Some studies show an increase in prolactin during the luteal phase. Halbreich found that women with PMS had higher prolactin levels than women who did not have PMS symptoms. Prolactin is produced by the pituitary gland and its job is to stimulate the development and growth of breast tissue. If the pituitary produces too much prolactin this will lead to breast tenderness, lumpiness and enlargement, and it may also alter the amount or balance of oestrogen and progesterone produced in the body, and affect mood.

PROSTAGLANDINS

A diet-related explanation concerns the role of prostaglandins in PMS. Prostaglandins are essential fatty acids (EFAs) that are made by the body. EFAs are nutritionally important to growth and health. The most important is linoleic acid, which is a polyunsaturated fatty acid found in cereals, pulses and vegetables. The richest sources are safflower-seed oil, evening primrose oil, sunflower, soya and corn oils. If you get most of the fat in your diet from animal fats, you may have a diet that is low in linoleic acid.

Prostaglandins act very much like hormones in that they, too, carry chemical messages around your system. When cells become damaged, prostaglandins are released into the blood, which cause inflammation and pain, drawing attention to the damage. This stimulates the body to take action to repair the situation. So, too much of these sorts of prostaglandins circulating in your blood would account for PMS symptoms such as pain and headaches.

Other prostaglandins, it is argued, have a regulatory effect on hormones such as oestrogen, progesterone and prolactin, keeping the right amount being produced. A deficiency in these would mean that there might be an imbalance in the levels of these hormones, so causing PMS symptoms. This explanation suggests that a diet lacking essential fatty acids that can be converted by the body into these prostaglandins would cause PMS. Some studies indicate that prostaglandins increase during the luteal phase and decline during menstruation as a normal and natural part of the menstrual cycle.

OPIOIDS

Another argument is that PMS is linked to opium-like substances made by the brain. These are actually called 'endogenous opioid peptides'. They are produced in your body to control your temperature, the way your bowels work, and whether and when you feel tired, hungry, happy and sad. Since some PMS symptoms mimic the

31

symptoms of narcotic withdrawal, such as nausea, cramps and depression, the theory that a lack of natural opioids leads to PMS has been advanced. Studies show that these opioids aren't only made in the brain but also in some way are affected by chemicals produced by your ovaries, so the levels may change throughout the menstrual cycle. If, in common with other ovarian hormones, they are at a low level in the premenstruum, this might explain a drop in mood. However, so far studies have failed to substantiate this.

BLOOD SUGAR

Another, but related, argument, and one advanced by Dalton, is that PMS has to do with low blood sugar. If you don't eat for some time the level of glucose or sugar in your blood drops. Glucose is the body's chief source of energy and is carried by the blood to all your tissues. Even though you may have a gap of several hours between meals, the level is normally kept within fairly narrow limits by the action of various hormones such as insulin and adrenaline. Glucose can be stored in the liver and muscles so that, if you go a long time between meals and your blood sugar level starts to drop, these reserves can be released.

The problem, of course, is that the release of adrenaline to stimulate this effect has its own side-effect of causing stress symptoms, making you jittery or tired. What may then happen is that you experience sweet cravings, and if you try to boost your level by eating sugar in the form, for instance, of chocolate, you can actually make the situation worse. This is because when you eat a high-sugar snack you get a very quick increase in the blood sugar level but this is followed immediately by a 'rebound' reaction, where the level falls. This sudden fall stimulates the release of more adrenaline which just starts the whole unpleasant cycle off again. This is why, once you start making up for hunger pangs with something like biscuits or chocolates, rather than satisfying you it makes you crave more. It is also suggested that when glucose is released from cells by adrenaline in this way, water takes its place and this is why you may suffer bloating.

'I binge eat. Every now and then I go mad for sweets and biscuits, chocolates most of all. I don't seem to be able to stop. When I really want something I just have to have it and I've been known to go down to the garage on the corner in my slippers in the middle of January at twelve at night to get a chocolate bar. The stupid thing is that even when I'm doing it I know that I'm not really enjoying it. It tastes really good, but half an hour or so I'll start up again. Give me chocolate at any other time in the month and I might have one, I might have two but then I've had enough and I don't want any more.'

NUTRITIONAL DEFICIENCIES

A further diet-related argument is that PMS is linked to vitamin or mineral deficiencies. Many PMS symptoms can be shown to be similar to the symptoms of various dietary deficiencies, such as a lack of vitamin B6, vitamin E, zinc, magnesium and others. It may seem highly unlikely that you could possibly be suffering from a lack of any important element in your food in modern society in the 1990s, especially if you are not going hungry. However, this is not as impossible as it seems. Modern diets are frequently lacking in essential dietary factors. If you eat a lot of convenience or processed foods and like 'fry ups', you may be horrified to find that essential vitamins are indeed not a part of your day-to-day eating.

EMOTIONAL FACTORS

Looking at the effects or influences of emotional states is probably the most contentious area to enter when trying to establish the causes of PMS. It's too close to the dismissive 'all in the mind' arguments, yet if we go too far down the line of insisting that PMS can *only* have physical causes, we are likely to miss out on something essential. One element vital to our understanding of the way our bodies work is the influence of mind on body, of body on mind. The actual mechanics of the way our minds and body relate are extremely complicated, but as an example consider the suggestion listed above under 'Opioids'.

When you feel an emotion it is the result of a signal or impulse carried in your brain by a chemical called a neurotransmitter. Your state of mind is the result of the delicate balance of your brain chemistry – a bit of this, a bit of that and the result is that you are sad, happy, angry or simply neutral. Your experiences in life, whether sad or happy things are happening to you, may be the trigger causing the production of these chemicals resulting in your emotional state. But it can happen the other way round – if your body is triggered into producing these chemicals, you'll then feel sad, happy etc. Which comes first can sometimes be a 'chicken or egg' question! So it is totally ridiculous to be dismissive about things being 'all in the mind'. You are not imagining it, or being neurotic or stupid, if you are undergoing an emotional state that an outsider feels doesn't fit your circumstances. Rather than being dismissive of your feelings, what needs to be done is to work out why your mind/body is reacting in this way.

So, without being in the least dismissive, it is useful to look at how emotional states, expectations and life experiences may affect the way you deal with and feel about your menstrual cycle.

Preparation for menstruation

There can be no doubt that it would be impossible to start your periods without having been prepared in some way for the event. The preparation can be an extremely positive one. In this situation a girl might have learned about the changes in her body and what they mean from a very early age, and heard her family talk freely and comfortably about periods for as long as she can remember. Periods may then be seen as a normal fact of life and in some ways rather exciting because they demonstrate a woman's ability to produce life itself.

The other extreme is the entirely negative view where open discussion of periods is taboo, and what the girl can pick up is that they are nasty, messy and painful, and something that sets women aside from the 'normal'. Sadly, in Western society, by the time you have your first period you are highly unlikely to have had a totally positive experience. You may have had some positive input, but what you have heard outside the home as well as experienced from your family is more likely to be somewhere along the line towards the negative one. This means that you will *expect* periods to be anything from a bother, to an embarrassing necessity, to a curse.

When your body, during puberty, changes from being one in which emotions and sensations are pretty similar from day to day, to one in which you experience a distinct alteration over the month, you are likely to associate discomfort and anxiety with this cycle. Everything else that happens then becomes linked in some way to your understanding that this change, this ebb and flow, is both abnormal and unusual, and the signal for something unpleasant. You are expecting it to cause distress. So is it any wonder that you interpret these changes as distressing?

'My grandmother used to get really annoyed with me

35

and my sister when we had our "off days". She said it was all nonsense and that we were making a lot of fuss about nothing. She was in her seventies then and that was around ten years ago. I asked her recently whether she had ever had problems with her periods, and she just laughed and laughed. She said periods weren't a problem, it was not having them that you had to watch out for. She said she was always pleased when she had a show because it was healthy to get all that bad blood out of you. But since she had ten children and lost a few more, she'd hardly had any periods to really talk about.'

Attitudes to menstruation

As already stated, there are several explanations for PMS that suggest it is caused by an unusual or abnormal physical state – with hormone levels being higher or lower, or some sort of deficiency. The problem is that studies frequently do not confirm this, finding that there is very little physical difference between women who do and women who do not report PMS. It's very tempting to point to a symptom or group of symptoms that are common to PMS sufferers, and claim that these prove a cause. For example, food cravings and poor diet could suggest the role of nutrition in causing and curing the syndrome. But a factor can really only unarguably be said to cause PMS if it is found in PMS sufferers and not in women who do not have this complaint. And so far, we haven't been able to prove any such single cause. Problems with food, for instance, are almost universal among women in Western society!

An argument could be therefore that the difference is not what physical state your body is in, but one of attitude. The differences are in the way you think and in the way you react. Any doctor or researcher proposing this is on pretty tricky ground because it seems to be suggesting that they think women who report PMS are therefore weak willed, while the ones who don't complain have a stiff upper lip, so it's all a question of pulling yourself together.

Doctors have a bad reputation for being unsympathetic and unhelpful with PMS. It's usually felt that this is because they are antagonistic towards women – doctors traditionally having been male. Those doctors who are female often behave in the same way since they were after all usually trained by men and are in what was always a very male-orientated profession.

There is, however, another explanation for doctors' apparent hostility towards women with PMS. This is that the medical profession is very much 'cure orientated'. Doctors are trained to see their job as identifying the cause of a problem and doing something about it. That's not just what they do, it's what they *are*. So when you present a doctor with a situation where they are powerless – where they don't know what's wrong, can't explain it and can't cure it – it can be a very unsettling situation for them. They can feel very threatened, very upset and angry. Unfortunately their anxiety is often directed at the patient. It's a rare doctor who can say 'Look, I haven't the foggiest why this is happening and I haven't got the power to do much about it.' Instead of accepting their own powerlessness, what the doctor will often do is blame you. It then becomes a case of 'It's your fault. You are making it up and it's not a real problem anyway.'

PMS *is* a real problem, but the exact nature of that reality is open for discussion. We shall be looking at that question in Chapter 5. Before that, however, we need to explore who suffers from PMS. This is the subject of Chapter 4.

4

Who has it?

There are a lot of myths about PMS and whether you may or may not be at risk of suffering from it. You may have heard or been told that:

- teenagers
- women who have had hysterectomies
- women who have been sterilised
- women who have not been pregnant
- women who have had babies
- women on the Pill

are all unlikely to suffer PMS, or even that they can't get this condition. Sadly, women from all these groups are well represented among PMS sufferers! However, as with most 'old Wives' tales', there is some grain of truth or reason for these myths, as will be explained.

Whether you *are* likely to suffer PMS *is* to a certain extent related to your age; or, rather, to your life stage. PMS can begin at any time after you have your first period. In spite of the belief that it is an older woman's condition, teenagers have been among the reported sufferers.

If you are too young to have periods or of an age when

your periods have stopped you won't have PMS. So girls who have not yet started their periods will not have PMS. Neither will women who have gone through the menopause and whose periods have finished. You may have headaches, moods, cramps and any other symptom that can also go with PMS – but it won't be PMS! PMS is strictly a condition that goes with having periods. Or, more properly, it is a condition that goes with having a menstrual cycle.

OVARIAN ACTIVITY

To refine it even further, it's a condition that goes hand in hand with having ovarian activity – that is, having working ovaries. So, teenagers at the very beginning of their menstrual cycles may not be prone to PMS because cycles in the first few months can be 'anovular', or without ovulation. When they do start to ovulate, the possibility to have PMS may come into play. At the other end of the scale, women who have had 'total' hysterectomies, in which their wombs have been removed so they don't bleed any more, can also still have PMS symptoms. This is because a so-called 'total' leaves their ovaries intact. As long as the ovaries go on working, the fact that there is no longer a womb to tell you what stage you are in the cycle by bleeding is neither here nor there. The ovaries will continue to measure out your menstrual cycle by producing their hormones, and you will continue to experience that ovarian activity in exactly the same way as you might have before losing your womb. An hysterectomy *will* remove PMS if it involves the surgical procedure that also takes away the ovaries. This is called a total hysterectomy with 'bi-lateral oophorectomy' (that is, both-sided removal of ovaries). In that case, and that case only, hysterectomy can be said to stop PMS.

'I've never really got on with the Pill, and the coil gave me heavy periods. So we used the condom for a couple of years which was all right but it's a bit of a bother. The GP said what did I think about sterilisation and I jumped at it. I must admit that one of the reasons I was so keen was that I've had PMS for years and it's a real bother. You get tired and moody, and you just don't know whether you're coming or going for at least a week every month. I don't know where I got the idea that sterilisation would do something about it. I think it was my mum's idea and I'd heard the same thing from other people. As it happened it didn't make the slightest bit of difference. If anything, I was worse off.'

There is a mistaken belief that sterilisation may lead to a reduction in PMS. This probably dates back to the days, several decades ago, when a hysterectomy would automatically have involved removal of the ovaries. Birth control was less effective then, so it might have been quite a relief to be free of the risks of further pregnancies, and free from unpleasant problems linked to periods. Word-of-mouth has kept all these things still associated in our minds, but sterilisation today will only stop PMS if you can no longer have children because your ovaries have been removed. The operation you would choose that cuts or blocks your fallopian tubes to prevent further pregnancies, leaves ovaries in place. So you would still be at risk of PMS. This is because your ovaries will still be acting to produce the hormones that run your menstrual cycle. As long as the menstrual cycle runs, so may PMS.

Just as PMS is absent before you begin to have periods and after you have finished having them it is also held at bay in the third part of life when you don't menstruate – when you are pregnant. However, pregnancy is not always good news as far as PMS is concerned. It's not true that women who have not yet been pregnant, or women who have had babies, don't get PMS. Plenty of women say PMS arrived with the first baby. And, for other women, their PMS became much worse after their first and even more unpleasant after subsequent pregnancies.

Another myth, challenged by many women with direct experience, is that women on the combined oral contraceptive pill, or the progestogen-only pill, do not suffer PMS. In spite of the fact that the combined contraceptive pill is often suggested as a treatment for PMS, women on the Pill may be just as likely to suffer PMS as women who are not on it. Indeed, when the Pill is tried as a treatment for PMS, it seems to worsen the condition or leave it un-affected as often as it helps.

It would seem that, potentially, all age groups, from teenagers to women just before menopause, can be suffer-ers of PMS.

One suggestion is that PMS may be associated with depression or other emotional difficulties. It may be reas-suring to know – and useful ammunition if any unsym-pathetic doctor seems to be suggesting otherwise! – that there is no evidence to support this. Women with no his-tory of depressive illness are just as likely to be among PMS sufferers as those who do have such a history.

What we *don't* know very much about is what character-istics may be shared by PMS sufferers. Are you more likely to have PMS if you are a stressed-out woman with a full-time job, or a serene, satisfied full-time mum (or a satisfied worker or a harassed mum)? What factors in your lifestyle or background have any bearing on PMS? Suffice to say that, at present, PMS seems to cross all race, class and age boundaries, in the Western world.

It *is*, however, found primarily in 'developed' countries and not reported as a problem in the emerging ones. Studies also suggest that the peak age for suffering PMS in our society would seem to be your thirties. Exactly why this may be so will be discussed in the next chapter.

5

Does PMS exist?

HISTORICAL EVIDENCE

Physicians through the ages, such as Galen who re-
searched, worked and wrote in second-century Rome, have
left us startlingly accurate descriptions of many diseases
and conditions. Women were often described as suffering
discomfort and emotional outbursts, and these were usually seen as somehow being linked to the menstrual cycle.
Semonides, in his essay on women written some 2600 years
ago, says:

> She has two different sorts of mood. One day she is all
> smiles and happiness ... there is no better wife ... nor
> prettier. Then another day there will be no living with
> her. You can't get within sight of or come near her or
> she flies into a rage and holds you at a distance like a
> bitch with pups, cantankerous and cross with all the
> world. The sea is like that also. Often it lies calm and
> innocent and still, then it will go wild and turbulent.
> This woman's disposition is just like the sea's since the
> sea's temper changes all the time.

One popular theory was that retained menstrual blood was somehow poisonous, an understandable deduction if you consider that what was being observed was that some women felt 'off' until their periods started and then felt better.

Something like PMS was first used as a defence in a murder trial in 1865, when Mary Harris was found not guilty of shooting her faithless lover by reason of her mental state. The defence at her trial had used medical evidence which described insanity associated with her menstrual periods. In 1931 the American physician Frank first described and defined what he called premenstrual tension. He suggested it was caused by inadequate female sex hormones. This was followed in 1934 by another American, Israel, who suggested that a defect in the luteinising stage of the menstrual cycle would result in a relative increase in progesterone over oestrogen, and so create premenstrual problems. However, it was not until 1953 that an article in the *British Medical Journal* by Greene and Dalton employed the name we now use – premenstrual syndrome.

The fact that PMS has only been described in the last hundred years could be simply a case of its not having been recognised. As with many situations or diseases, once it becomes a matter of public debate, many people feel able to come out and say that this is their problem, too. You may have the idea that PMS, like sexual abuse or post-natal depression, has only appeared in the twentieth century, because they were so little talked about before. They all seem to be conditions of our times. There is a difference, however. Some things, such as sexual abuse, have always been there, but were hidden behind a conspiracy of silence. Once this silence is broken, you get a flood of those able to bring their story into the light. There is a case to be made, however, for saying that the reason PMS has become a modern disease, is because it is a modern disease. The combination of conditions that produce it may not have been present in earlier times.

PERIODS TODAY

You need to remember that our great-grandmothers had far fewer periods than we do. They experienced their first bleed – the menarche – later than we do now, and the menopause and their last periods came earlier. In between, they had babies instead of periods!

A woman in the West today will have her first period at around 12 and her last in her fifties. In between, she will have two-point-four children and some four hundred periods. In contrast, great-grandmother had several children who survived to adulthood, several who died in childhood and may even have had several miscarriages. She breastfed for up to a year, or even more, each time. As a result she probably only had 35 periods in her lifetime. Women in societies today, in the emerging countries, in which the same patterns of childbearing are found, do not appear to have a problem with PMS.

'My mother was a medical student in South Africa and she did some work in the townships. I always remember something she told me when I had a particularly bad period one month, when I was a teenager. She said she'd had this one woman who came to her, who was terrified she was dying and something was terribly wrong with her. She was bleeding, and my mother was all for doing tests and rushing her off for a transfusion when an experienced doctor pointed out the woman was having a period. The reason why it was so frightening and confusing was that she was 30 or so and it was the first time she'd ever had a period. She'd been pregnant or breastfeeding ever since puberty.'

PMS seems to be a luxury only 'civilised' cultures can afford. It would seem not only to be a condition of the menstrual cycle, but also one related to the number and type of cycles you experience.

DEFINING PMS

One of the main reasons for much of the argument about PMS is that no one can come up with a definition of what it is that everyone agrees with. It's often pointed out that most of the studies on PMS come up with conflicting findings. A treatment that one study shows to be extremely effective will do little or nothing in another. Part of the problem, however, could be that each study may actually be looking at different things. For instance, let us say you define PMS as a condition in which women suffer severely from a specified number of symptoms, and try to see whether a particular therapy helps at all. You would necessarily have very different results than if you said PMS is a condition in which various symptoms occurred during a particular time period, and looked to see if another therapy helped with these. Similarly, you are going to come up with different findings if you make that time period four days before a period starts and four days afterwards, than if you decide it has to be five days before and two days afterwards. In each of these cases, you are looking at a different picture, which may therefore have different reasons for what is happening. You are rather hedging your bets if you declare you have the definitive, fail-safe treatment for 'true' PMS because you can then always argue that anyone taking your particular therapy who doesn't improve must quite clearly not be a 'true' PMS sufferer!

There is no doubt that PMS is a touchy issue, and not just for those who experience it. It would seem that there are plenty of vested interests in confirming or denying its very existence. There is a lot of money to be made, in both conventional and alternative medicine, in deciding exactly what is PMS and what causes it, and then in offering the 'cure'. But it is not just monetary gain here; it is also a professional one. Because if it is a disease that doctors can cure this puts the medical profession in a position of power over women. Gender politics are at stake too, because if you accept the idea that a woman's monthly cycle almost inevitably leads to physical and emotional disturbance, you may also be saying that women are therefore less re-liable and effective, and more vulnerable than their male counterparts.

Dalton argues that women suffer an increased incidence of crime and alcoholism, school problems, sickness at work, accidents and hospital admissions in the week before menstruation, and that PMS is responsible. How-ever, researchers who have done controlled studies say there is no significant variation in the physical skills or emotional stability of women associated with their menstrual cycles. They say that social behaviour, such as criminal or self-destructive acts, are subject to a bias when self-reported. That is, when you only base your theories on people who come forward, you are likely to get a skewed result. In a controlled study, this effect disappears.

It is interesting to note that in one study a group of women were convinced that the researchers could accur-ately pinpoint whereabouts they were in their menstrual cycle. Half were told they were premenstrual, the other half that they were mid-way between periods. All were actually six or seven days from their periods, yet the 'pre-menstrual' group reported significantly higher levels of pain, water retention and a greater change of eating pat-terns than the others. In another study, girls who had not yet started having periods were found to agree with the statements 'Girls are grouchy just before a period' and

'Girls are more likely to get upset and nervous when they menstruate than when they don't menstruate'. The moral? We are not stupid, but never underestimate the power of expectation, anticipation and suggestion!

If you want to test this for yourself, make your partner or your friend a cup of coffee. Casually tell them several times you are making tea and hand them the cup saying 'Here's your tea'. See how long it takes them to notice they are drinking coffee not tea. Some will find, when you question them afterwards, that their expectation was so powerful that they genuinely tasted a different beverage from the one you had given them.

You can see PMS as a purely medical dilemma. If it is an abnormal condition or set of conditions, then the way to deal with it is to return the woman to normality by changing or curing either the way this syndrome makes itself felt – the symptoms – or tackling the original cause. Some of the treatments offered attempt to deal with symptoms, while some try to pinpoint the cause and deal with that. But there is a further route and this involves looking at the situation in an entirely different way.

Consider the situation. We are saying that each month women may experience a range of changes. Their emotions, their bodies and sense of well being may alter. These changes are perceived as unpleasant and therefore unacceptable. But what if it is not the changes so much as the expectation that is at fault?

IS PMS 'NORMAL'?

It's possible that PMS is not really an abnormal condition at all. Quite a few studies have found that when you compare PMS to non-PMS women the two groups actually show no physical differences at all. Frequently what they appear to be experiencing is very similar. The only difference is that those who say they have unpleasant symptoms they ascribe to PMS find what they experience to be intolerable. What is different is not what happens during their menstrual cycles but how they react to or cope with the changes related to their menstrual cycles.

It could be argued that, rather than being an actual condition, PMS is a useful umbrella or a sort of entrance ticket. If you are feeling tired, distressed, angry or at the end of your tether, you may still find it quite difficult to go to your doctor, or anyone else, and ask for help. If you go in and say you have PMS, even with an unsympathetic GP, you may at least feel that you have a valid reason for claiming some time and attention.

Although PMS can occur at any age, peak incidence appears to be in women in their early and mid thirties. This is a time in the majority of women's lives when you are likely to have an enormous amount on your plates. Most women at that point have young children and a home to look after. You may also have a part-time or a full-time job. It's a time when you may be putting a lot of time and effort into your family, and have less energy, or thought, to look after yourself. You may be spending a lot of time helping everyone else have friends and a social life, but letting your own go by the board. It's the very time when you may be feeling as if you are caring for everyone else and no one is caring for you. If you are single and/or without children, this in itself may put some form of pressure on you, either because of other people's disappointment or expectations of your own.

Studies looking at marital satisfaction also suggest it may be the time in your life when happiness could be at a low point. All the advantages or benefits of marriage and family may at this time be outweighed by the drawbacks. The honeymoon is well and truly over. If you have children they may have reached the stage where they are the most work and the least fun. If you are on your own from choice or chance, it's a time when you may feel time is passing you by and you may have regrets. But demanding some care and attention for yourself may be difficult, which is where PMS may come in. PMS is a less hurtful or frightening explanation to those around you, and to yourself, of your strong and painful feelings. Going to a doctor and asking for a diagnosis of PMS may be a legitimate way of demanding some help. Sadly, it's also an effective way of not perhaps examining more painful explanations for your feelings.

Women are brought up in this society to feel that anger and disagreements are unfeminine. Men can shout and fight, and although nobody likes raised voices this is still behaviour that is acceptable because it is appropriate. 'Boys will be boys' after all. But if a little girl raises her voice, and especially if she makes a fist and hits out, she will get the worst of all punishments – disapproval. It's just 'not done' for a woman or a girl to behave like that, and she quickly learns that if she is to be acceptable to men and other women she must be 'nice'.

In the film *The Stepford Wives*, the heroine was horrified to discover that the men in the idyllic small town she and her husband moved to were replacing their flesh and blood wives with 'perfect' automata. Many women can be forgiven for thinking that these robotic stereotypes are every man's fantasy of what a woman should be. It's hardly surprising that most of us would like to rebel against this, but the fear is that we would be accused of being bitchy, neurotic or unfeminine. Once a month, however, we have the perfect excuse for being angry and uncooperative – 'It's not me, it's the PMS talking.'

'My parents really lost control of me when I was a teenager. I used to have these dreadful fits of temper and I've had bad PMS which lasted into my twenties. I really did grow up with this message that raising your voice was a terrible thing to do. Nobody else did it in my family. My boyfriend didn't like it either. He was not the sort of person you could have an argument with. It was just like with my parents, that all sorts of things would be going on under the surface but you wouldn't talk about it. I really did feel this pressure to 'be nice'. And when I didn't feel nice, well that was because I was having a bad month with the PMS.'

There are a lot of things to be angry about. Even if you are lucky enough to be brought up in a loving and accepting family, and grow up to make happy and satisfying relationships, it's still an unfair world out there. There are times when you would have every right to want to express nasty, messy, negative emotions. But if you are not allowed to express them, if you have been brought up to feel that having them at all somehow means you are a failure, where is that anger going to go? Suppressing anger doesn't make it go away. Suppressed anger goes underground and what happens then is that it turns on you. If you don't recognise it, if you don't own it, it's likely to turn up in all sorts of uncomfortable ways – as depression, as feelings of self-disgust, as headaches. Stress-related illnesses are not only emotional, either. Stress leads to heart attacks and it is not unreasonable to suggest that it may lead to PMS.

BEING A WOMAN IN A MAN'S WORLD

PMS may be a reaction to the problems of being a woman in a male-oriented world. Suppressed anger and dissatisfaction may culminate in or emerge as PMS symptoms for several reasons. One is that the menstrual cycle is, after all, a continual reminder that you are female, with all the constraints and the negative image that this culture imposes upon you. There are still plenty of myths that paint menstruation as an unpleasant and undesirable state. A World Health Organisation Study (WHO 1983) found that in the UK 10 per cent of respondents said that women should avoid bathing during a period, 5 per cent thought a woman shouldn't wash her hair, 7 per cent thought menstruation was dirty and like a sickness, and 54 per cent believed sex should be avoided during menstruation. It would hardly be surprising then that your unconscious mind would react to the impending signals that your period is due. But it's also a time in which you have been given permission to offload all those 'unfeminine' behaviour patterns, a time when you can shout and scream without being punished because you can always claim that it wasn't you, it was the PMS talking.

This is not the same as saying that PMS is neurotic or imagined. Put anyone in an unnatural or intolerable situation, with conflicting demands, and they will react in some way. What is wrong is not women, but the expectations society puts on us.

When we are experiencing a problem it can be enormously reassuring to have a proper label for it. There are two reasons for this. One is that if we can label it the chances are that we can do something about it. The second is that if there is a label for it we are blameless. The sad fact is that we still have an attitude to physical symptoms that have a physical cause which is different from the attitude we have towards emotional difficulties. In this atmosphere, physical difficulties are seen to be 'good'. They are beyond your control, they exist and it's not your fault if you have them. Emotional difficulties, on the other hand, are seen to be 'bad'. They are a sign that you are neurotic, lazy, hysterical or malingering – that you are 'female'! But the fact is that if PMS does have an emotional cause, as a single cause or as one of several causes, it does not make your problem any less real. Nor does it mean you can do nothing about it. Emotional difficulties can be dealt with. You might even say they can sometimes be dealt with more easily than physical ones, because having an emotional problem puts much of the power to do something about it in your own hands, not the hands of a doctor.

'I changed doctors three times trying to find a cure for my PMS. Each said they couldn't find anything physically wrong with me and I'd get so angry that they were telling me it was all in my mind. It affected our marriage and got so bad that my husband went to live with his sister for a few weeks. She and her husband had been to Relate, and she persuaded Bob to make me go along with him. I didn't want to go and I really hated the first few times we saw a woman there. What made a difference was that she was so matter of fact and sympathetic, and got me to understand that having an emotional problem wasn't sick or silly, or even unusual. The way she put it was that what we didn't want was to have a label stuck on us, but we could take the help without taking the label. So we had counselling for our marriage, but it was for my PMS too. And it wasn't her doing it to us, it was us doing it for ourselves and that's what made all the difference.'

Maybe the core of the problem is that we live in a society which is male oriented. Men are in positions of power both politically and socially; men are in the main the doctors, writers, historians and illustrators of society. Open a history book, walk through an art gallery or read a medical text and with very few exceptions the picture you see of *human*kind is actually that of *man*kind. But men and women are very different.

The human race reproduces by using two sexes. One sex is required to contribute its genes through a package assimilated by the other. The male of the species produces its genetic material continually because its only job is to make that contribution. The female of the species has three jobs – to contribute genes, to carry and birth offspring, and to feed it. With only one job to do the male body is fairly static. Sperm is produced continually and although individual sperm may proceed from its creation to its final maturation over a period of several weeks within the body, because the process is continual the body itself is unchanging.

The female body has a very different job and so has to go about it in another way. Women go through cycles as the body readies itself to bring an egg to maturation, to make it available for conception and to implant that egg if fertilisation happens. The body then sustains new life, brings it to maturation and when it is born provides sustenance. If fertilisation doesn't occur, the female body goes on to prepare itself for another chance.

Ebb and flow, change and difference are the stuff of the female body and the female experience. The problem is that we live in a culture that says alteration is abnormal and that stability is the only acceptable norm. To be mystical for a moment, we no longer worship the moon goddess, who through every month presents a different face to the world, but a patriarchal god, who insists that you must be unvarying or that there is something wrong with you. But there is nothing wrong with us when our bodies, and our emotions, travel along that roller coaster each month. The only 'abnormality' lies in a society that keeps telling us our experience is out of the ordinary!

Up to puberty, the female body is in line with the male body, in that it doesn't change from month to month. With puberty come external changes in both. But, in addition, in the female body comes a change that is not seen as 'normal' in the world at large – the beginning of a dramatic fluctuation every month. It starts, for women in the

Western world, around the age of 12 and goes on occurring every month for the next 40 years or so.

One consequence of beginning to have your periods at around the age of 12 and not having a pregnancy until at the earliest your late teens, or more likely your middle twenties, is that you very quickly become habituated to the switchback of the menstrual cycle. Each month your body goes through quite a dramatic rise and fall, and alteration of various hormonal levels. You will know how easy it is to fall into a routine – like wearing a groove into the carpet because every day you take the same steps from bedroom to bathroom. You may be emotionally used to the fact that once a month you have a period, but your body physically becomes accustomed to that fact too. In a sense, because modern women start early, go on having periods so late, and have so many periods, our reaction to this monthly ebb and flow may also become exaggerated. This means that often, even if you break up your routine by using medication to prevent the ovaries working, such as going on the Pill, your brain still expects the long-accustomed rhythm, and triggers the same emotional and physical symptoms that you recognise and suffer as PMS.

But if PMS is not abnormal or unusual, why do so many of us experience it as unpleasant? Surely evolution would not have produced such a flawed design – a body that routinely causes discomfort? Perhaps there is a very good reason for PMS.

The function of any successful animal is to breed and have children – it's what our bodies are designed for. So each month you don't fall pregnant is, in the natural sense, a missed chance. Just as sexual pleasure is likely to be 'the carrot' to get you to engage in sexual intercourse so you can perpetuate the species, so the unpleasant sensations of PMS may be 'the stick' for not falling pregnant. The unpleasant sensations of PMS begin with and are triggered by the hormonal changes that signal fertilisation has not occurred. And they end when your body begins to prepare for another try.

One doctor, Parlee, has said that the assessment of PMS is less the measure of individual behaviour than of socially shared belief. In other words, every woman undergoes a series of changes each month – it goes with the territory. But considering these changes as worrying and abnormal makes them intolerable, and it is society and its attitudes to being a woman in general, and menstruation in particular, that makes them so.

There can be no doubt that many women experience PMS. Exactly what it is and why it happens is open for debate, however. One, perhaps practical, approach is to accept the idea that PMS has a host of causes, rather than one, simple, cause. If it is not so much a disease but a response to normal events, then we have to accept that looking to outsiders, whether doctors or other helpers, for a cure as such may not produce what we want. Each person who has symptoms is more likely to find something, or things, which work if they look for their own, individual, answer. Rather than a pill or other specific treatment, this may be anything that gives you a feeling of being healthy and in control. Later in the book, we will be looking at a wide range of suggested treatments.

Before that, it may be helpful to decide whether PMS is your problem. Whether you decide you have PMS or not, putting your symptoms under the spotlight is bound to be a useful exercise. In the next chapter we shall be looking at ways to determine whether or not your problem is linked to or caused by your menstrual cycle, or your response to it.

6

Do I have it?

KEEPING A MENSTRUAL DIARY

If you are experiencing physical or emotional changes that seem unacceptable or intolerable to you, before you go any further you need to work out whether these could be grouped under the heading PMS. Your own doctor may be able to help you, but even before you make an appointment at your surgery, you need a clearer picture of what is going on. The only way you are going to be able to do this is to keep a menstrual diary.

To make a diagnosis of PMS there has to be some sort of a pattern in the symptoms you experience. You can only see if this pattern exists if you keep a day-to-day note of your physical and emotional feelings and do so for at least three, and preferably six, menstrual cycles. You may find it most helpful to have a preliminary month noting down and taking account of the symptoms that bother you. Are these physical, such as headaches, nausea, joint aches, breast tenderness or a feeling of being bloated? Are they emotional changes, such as irritableness, difficulties with concentration, anger or depression? Or are they a combination of the physical and the emotional? After a month, pick a number of symptoms that you feel to be the most important. You may choose three or four, or as many as six. If you are monitoring what happens in your body and in your mind over a month you may also note some changes that you might not exactly call 'symptoms' because you may not experience them as particularly bothersome. One may be that you go to the loo to pass water more or less often on particular days in your cycle. Another could be that instead of actually having cravings for certain types of food you do, however, get a taste for pasta or having an extra spoon of sugar in your coffee at particular times of the month.

'I went to see my doctor in a terrible state. I'd been having PMS for a couple of years but it's been getting particularly bad over the last few months. He said before he could do anything I'd have to keep a diary. He said he wanted to help but that I should trust him and this was the right way to go about it. He was right because the worst thing of all was that it just used to get on top of me. I didn't want to keep the diary because I didn't know where I was going to start. I just couldn't see a way of making any sense of it. He went through this chart with me and just by thinking what the main problems were it started to get it in a sort of focus. When I kept the diary it was as if I was putting things in pigeon holes and that stopped it spilling out all over the place. When I was writing it down it started to show that I really only had these symptoms for about 8 days every month, not just about 28 days which was the way I'd seen it. When I could see on paper that I felt OK on more days that I felt bad I found I could brace myself for the bad days better. And then, of course, when I went back with the diary written up and we could see what was wrong, and when it happened, he started treating me.'

Using a diary or calendar, or the chart we print here, keep track of the changes you experience. Start off by filling in the key opposite. Under 'symptoms', list those you want to keep track of and the symbol you will use to identify it. For instance, you could use 'H' for headache, 'BT' for breast tenderness and 'I' for irritability. Then, under 'body changes', list things that seem different even if you are not sure they are unpleasant enough to constitute a symptom or not. On the days you pass more water than usual you could put 'W+' and on those where you pass less you might put 'W−'. If you have food cravings, list these as 'C' with a second smaller symbol to indicate the type of food you want. For example 'Cs' could indicate a craving for sweet things and 'Cc' could be for carbohydrates such as pasta or bread. You may also like to put in some indication of the severity of your symptoms. Take it as read that your base line is symptoms that are uncomfortable to the point of being unacceptable and then add a minus if you notice them but they are not too bad, a plus if they are particularly unpleasant and even a double plus if they are so bad you're suffering intolerably.

Keep your Symptom Chart by your bedside and fill it in each night as you go to bed. If you feel any of these symptoms have been definitely present during the day, mark them on the chart. Put a line through the day if you haven't had any symptoms. That way you will be certain later that it wasn't just because you had forgotten to make an entry! Mark the day on which your period begins and each day that you have bleeding. The best way of doing this is with a red dot or by colouring in the spaces on the chart.

Key to Your Symptoms

Symptoms	Symbol	Body Changes

Symptom Chart

	Month 1	Month 2	Month 3	Month 4	Month 5	Month 6
1						
2						
3						
4						
5						
6						
7						
8						
9						

	Month 1	Month 2	Month 3	Month 4	Month 5	Month 6
10						
11						
12						
13						
14						
15						
16						
17						
18						
19						
20						
21						
22						
23						
24						
25						
26						

	Month 1	Month 2	Month 3	Month 4	Month 5	Month 6
27						
28						
29						
30						
31						

Total honesty is obviously very important. You may find it very tempting after the first month or so to forget certain days or exaggerate your feelings on another, particularly if the pattern beginning to emerge doesn't immediately suggest PMS. If you are having a bad time or feel you need help it may be very tempting for you to want this to be PMS. But bending your experiences in order to create such a diagnosis is not going to help if it's not PMS you're experiencing. Only an accurate record will help you and your doctor find out what is wrong.

Getting a clear picture of what is happening is obviously vital if you are to do anything about it. Once you can see the pattern of the difficulties you are experiencing you, on your own and in partnership with your doctor, can set about doing something about it. Deciding you have PMS without keeping a proper menstrual diary for a sufficient length of time isn't going to get you anywhere, and your doctor won't be able to help without pretty clear evidence. Our memories are not always accurate, so even though you may be convinced that your symptoms come like clockwork just before your period, it is an important discipline to keep a diary for a few months.

Keeping a menstrual diary may have another useful

feature. One of the distressing aspects of PMS is the feeling of being at the mercy of what is happening to you, of being confused and overwhelmed by your body, and your emotions no longer being in your control. Just the act of keeping your diary puts you back in some sort of control. By organising information, you also start to organise yourself, and this can be very reassuring.

If you haven't started keeping a diary before you see your doctor for the first time you are going to have to do so before he or she can offer you some treatment anyway, so it's worth starting now.

If you find the pattern that emerges from your chart does not suggest PMS, don't despair. The picture that may emerge may be just as useful to enable you and your doctor to find out what other diagnosis can be made.

'I was sure the symptoms I was having only came in the week before my period. I wasn't far wrong with that because that was when they mostly came. But when I started writing them down every time it happened I saw it came at other times as well and it didn't get better when my periods started, sometimes it got worse. I went and saw my doctor and he suggested I might have endometriosis.'

WHAT ELSE COULD IT BE?

Dysmenorrhoea

Dysmenorrhoea is the formal medical name for painful periods. It's either primary dysmenorrhoea, which means you've had painful periods from when you first started having periods, or it's secondary dysmenorrhoea, which means that your periods became painful some time afterwards. In both cases dysmenorrhoea is a description rather than a diagnosis. That is, the period pain is usually caused by something, and you and your doctor may want to find out what this is. Primary dysmenorrhoea usually comes in one of two forms – spasmodic or congestive.

Spasmodic dysmenorrhoea is when you get severe, gripping pains that strike just before your period or when it begins and can continue until bleeding stops. The cramps are centred in the uterus and affect the groin area, and the inside of the thighs, radiating outwards. Spasmodic dysmenorrhoea is also often accompanied by feelings of nausea and sometimes by headaches. Women who suffer from spasmodic dysmenorrhoea often find it becomes less or clears up altogether once they've had a pregnancy.

Keeping in mind that dysmenorrhoea is a description rather than a diagnosis, 'congestive dysmenorrhoea' may actually be another way of describing PMS. This is period pain that starts some days before a period begins. Instead of acute pain there is a dull, dragging ache which gradually worsens until the first day of bleeding when it recedes quickly or immediately. Women with congestive dysmenorrhoea are likely to have tender and swollen breasts, a bloated tummy, and may find that joints ache, fingers and feet swell, they have headaches, sinus problems, acne, are clumsy, have difficulty sleeping and are irritable. As soon as a period begins a weight is lifted and the symptoms disappear. Don't forget that understanding what is going wrong and exactly how to fix it in the human body is not as easy as diagnosing a fault and fixing it in a car engine. A lot of the time doctors put a label on a set of symptoms purely to make themselves feel better and to give them a start point for treatment. The reason PMS and congestive dysmenorrhoea are not said to be the same thing is that with congestive dysmenorrhoea the symptoms can occur for as long as two weeks before a period begins.

Secondary dysmenorrhoea is when period pains develop after a history of normal periods. Again, the name is a description of the result rather than a diagnosis of the reason. The cause could be emotional or a medical condition such as fibroids, tumours, endometriosis (see below), PID (see below) or polyps.

Mittelschmerz

If you suffered from a few days of uncomfortable, gripping pain and were a bit vague about when it occurred, but knew it was some time before your period began and distinct from it, you may mistake this for a form of premenstrual discomfort. The condition may however be Mittelschmerz or 'middle pain'. This actually occurs around the time of ovulation, 12 to 16 days before your next period begins. At ovulation the follicle, or area in your ovary that contains an egg, ruptures or breaks open, throwing out the egg which is then carried down the fallopian tube towards the uterus. Some women actually experience aching or sharp pain when this happens and may pass a few drops of blood at the same time, which is what could cause confusion about the exact timing in the month when it happens. Keeping a menstrual diary would tell you whether you had period pain or Mittelschmerz.

Endometriosis

Endometriosis is a condition that can produce many symptoms similar to those experienced with PMS. Pain, particularly before a period, depression, tiredness, difficulties in passing urine and bowel upsets are all common symptoms. Endometriosis is a condition in which tissue that is normally only found in the lining of the womb grows in other places. Endometrial tissue is designed to be the thick, cushioning lining rich in blood vessels in which a fertilised egg embeds itself. Endometrial tissue is triggered by hormonal changes each month to grow and then to be shed if a pregnancy doesn't occur. This is fine if the tissue lines the womb since, as it comes away, it can flow out of the body through the channel from the uterus to the vagina. However, endometriosis occurs when this tissue is found in other places such as inside the walls of the uterus, on the outside of the uterus or on ovaries, inside the pelvic cavity, on ligaments, on the outside of the bowel, or indeed inside the walls of the bowel or the walls of the pelvic cavity.

Endometriotic deposits thicken and then shed blood following the monthly cycle, and this is quite damaging in its effects. Blood in the wrong place is an irritant and the parts of the body surrounding these deposits may become inflamed. Large cysts may form which can press painfully on surrounding organs, and scar tissue may grow that can stick ligaments and organs together. Some symptoms of endometriosis may follow a monthly cycle. Discomfort, and thus tiredness and depression, may be particularly acute just before a period. However, the resolution and absence of symptoms soon after a period begins, which is a characteristic of PMS, will not be there for endometriosis.

Menopause

On the surface you would think it would be difficult to confuse menopause with PMS. After all, menopause is when your periods start decreasing until they stop, while PMS goes hand in hand with ongoing menstrual cycles. But it's easy to see how you may suspect PMS, when in fact what is happening is that you are approaching menopause. This is because PMS can get worse or indeed only worsen to the point at which you complain about it as you get older. If you go to your doctor with symptoms such as joint pains, depression, anxiety and forgetfulness, with an increased urge to pass water or cystitis, and you are over the age of 40, menopause may actually be the cause. Don't discount the possibility of it being the menopause rather than PMS even if you are under 40. Very early or premature menopause is by no means rare and you will certainly need advice from your doctor if this is what is happening rather than PMS.

Chronic PID

Pelvic inflammatory disease or PID is a widespread infection in the reproductive and pelvic organs. It can have a variety of causes and can be acute, where you may experience fever, discharge and sudden pain, or chronic. When it's chronic you may have some discharge, pain and general ill-health, but at a grumbling level that may not alert you to the fact that you need to see a doctor and have treatment. Chronic PID can flare up and die down, and may indeed become worse just before a period begins.

The IUD

Women who have had an IUD inserted may find that their periods become heavier or more painful. It sounds rather unlikely that anyone who has had an IUD inserted may not realise that it could be associated with a change in the patterns of their periods or their physical reactions. If cramps and discomfort don't occur immediately but worsen gradually some time after you have otherwise satisfactorily started using this form of contraception, you may not make this link.

Ill-health

Many symptoms that might lead to a diagnosis of PMS can equally be indicative of a range of illnesses or worrying conditions. You don't have to be neurotic or a hypochondriac to want to check out, with your doctor's help, anything that is a result of your feeling below par. Any persistent discomfort should be explored. The occasional headache, gut twinge or back strain is quite obviously just a part of life and you are worrying unnecessarily if you rush to the doctor every time you feel slightly under the weather. But if, in the course of every month, you have regular headaches, regular stomach pains or regular back pains, you should find out why it's happening. It may be PMS, or it may be diabetes, a kidney condition or even that you need glasses.

Medical treatment

A surprising number of conditions are 'iatrogenic' which means a condition that results from medical treatment – in other words, a side effect. Doctors and medicine labels aren't always able to warn you fully of what may happen to you. If you develop any condition or set of uncomfortable symptoms, either for the first time or in a more intense form that previously, the first thing you should always do is consider what has recently changed in your life. If you started any form of medical treatment recently, or have been under treatment for some time that only recently might have reached its full effects, you should consider whether this has played a part in what you are experiencing.

Emotional problems

As already outlined in Chapter 5, it may be difficult to separate complex feelings that have their origin in a wide range of causes from emotional to those triggered purely by bodily reactions. It would be understandable that you might react with irritation to any suggestion that your physical feelings are 'all in the mind'. It is always more satisfactory to feel that an unpleasant condition may be physical in origin, if for no other reason than the belief that if it has a physical cause it will respond easily to physical therapy. You may think that if you can establish that your depression is caused by PMS it can be cured by merely taking a pill. But it has to be more complex than that, and it is not dismissive to suggest that unpleasant cyclical symptoms may have their origin in your emotions, and that the best way of dealing with them is to explore, understand and deal with those very emotions.

Perceptions and lifestyle

Again, as already outlined in Chapter 5, whether or not you may be defined as having PMS could have a lot to do with both your expectations and the way you live. If you expect youself to remain unchanging from day to day, puberty would be a bit of a shock. The fact is that women's bodies and our emotions climb on to a roller-coaster from that time. Alterations will take place, and if you don't expect this or learn to understand and accept it, you may well find yourself reacting to normal change as if it were the onset of a problem. What may need looking at is not your body, but your understanding and appreciation of it. If your expectations are unrealistic, what can happen is that your response to something that is perfectly natural becomes disproportionate. An increase in the size and sensitivity, and a change in texture of breast tissue which one woman may see as 'just something that happens every month', another may fear as a sign of trouble. This is not to say that the second woman is being stupid, over-reacting or being neurotic. The unexpected is always frightening, but the problem is that we don't know about or expect these changes.

If you don't expect it, it can take you by surprise, but there is another way that expectations can inform your reaction. Simply by seeing periods and menstrual change as unpleasant and a chore magnifies their effects. If you grow up knowing periods as 'the curse' they will fulfil your expectations. And it may not be your own expectations alone that inform this. The attitudes of your parents, teachers, friends and your sexual partner all have an effect on the way you deal with your cyclical change.

Not understanding your own limits can also affect the way you experience your menstrual cycle. What you eat, whether you drink too much, smoke at all and how much exercise you take, can all have a dramatic effect on your well being. If you have an immensely stressful life with the demands of being all things to all people in your family, social circle and at work, it may be hardly surprising that you often feel tired, irritable and aching. It's not PMS that is making you feel so awful, it's your lifestyle! Whether PMS is your problem or not, some of the suggestions in Chapter 10 could be very helpful to you. But if you are on the way to deciding whether PMS is your problem or not, before we look at treatments it might first be useful to consider why PMS isn't only your problem. How the men you come into contact with may help you, or compound your difficulties, how they may be feeling and how their attitudes affect you, is the theme of Chapter 7.

7

PMS and the men in your life

There is a lot to be said for the theory that men fear
women's power. That sounds rather odd because no one
will deny the fact that most men are stronger than most
women. Your average man is taller, heavier and bigger
than your average woman. There are, of course, fast,
strong and large women – you only have to watch
women's sport to know that many women could trounce
many men in the arena. But differences in bone structure
and muscle composition mean that the top-level men
will always beat top-level women in any sport that
simply needs strength or speed. And when it comes to
power and domination, strength and speed tend to be
what matters.

EARLY HISTORY

But women have a power that from the beginning of time
men have envied and struggled to come to terms with.
This is that women have babies. All men start their lives
emerging from a woman's body. All men spend their

earliest days dependent on a woman. And all men have their first allegiance and love to a woman. Gratitude, awe and affection are one response to this; jealousy, fear and anger, and a desire to denigrate the very thing that holds you in thrall is another.

There is evidence to suggest that centuries ago men and women held positions in society different from those they hold now. It's possible that men and women were ignorant of the role men played in pregnancy, and women were felt to have the sole power to produce life. That ability alone gave them the position of 'wise women'. But it's also been suggested that in many cultures women had a greater role in the maintenance of social order than we traditionally record. We are used to learning about men as the elders, lawmakers and leaders of early communities. We are used to hearing about 'man the hunter' and of thinking that men brought home the bacon – or the antelope – to feed the family. An alternative view is that the majority of sustenance was provided from foraging – nuts, grains, roots and fruit – and that this was done by the women. Animal protein came to acquire a status because the bigger, stronger and faster men insisted that their contribution should be given high priority, but not because it was actually the most important. It's also possible that women actually did most of the running of the household and village. The men, however, took the credit.

Somewhere along the line a gigantic con trick was worked. The very things that made women powerful, admired and envied were re-defined as the marks of shame and discomfort. The ability to bleed without a wound, and without experiencing any harm, was made a source of shame and embarrassment. Menstruation became a taboo, and was seen as dirty and even polluting. Pregnancy and childbirth became events not to celebrate in themselves but only to be celebrated in certain circumstances. Children

71

became possessions owned by men and pregnancy was a good thing only if it occurred within a union sanctioned by Church and State.

The main difficulty in getting men to come to terms with the effects of PMS is that history and perceived wisdom work against us. We largely have a past where man has been the dominant figure and therefore the 'norm'. Since men's bodies are essentially static, except for the one major upheaval of puberty, it is very easy for them to consider the monthly switchback changes in the woman's body as being irrational, or even sick or neurotic.

It is a rather chicken-and-egg situation in that it's very difficult to point a finger at exactly how and when this started, and thus get off the merry-go-round. Our earliest experiences are likely to be of menstruation being a taboo subject. If you are lucky you will grow up in a home where this is not so, but even if you can talk freely at home, once you go outside, you will find the pressure is on to avoid the subject. More often sex and periods will be subjects not talked about openly in your family.

The fact that periods and 'that time of the month' are a bit of a mystery makes them both frightening and intriguing. When you do ask questions or hear things, you are likely to gather, openly and under the surface, that periods are 'not nice', painful and dirty. It's very hard for a young boy to grow up seeing menstruation as anything other than puzzling, distasteful and rather alarming. It's hardly surprising that when faced with anything inexplicable in the emotional responses of the women he deals with, or any response he would rather not acknowledge, he's likely to fall back on the excuse, 'Well I couldn't understand it even if I tried. It's nothing to do with me – it's female problems'. When you are excluded from a club, or embarrassed by what a closed group of people are discussing, what's the normal, human reaction? It's to say 'What a lot of stuff and nonsense, I didn't want to join in anyway!'

HIS FEARS AND FANTASIES

The beliefs of all the men you come into contact with, whether your partner, work colleagues or members of your family, will have a huge influence on how you see yourself and on how much self-assurance you can muster when dealing with any problems relating to your PMS. It will help you to understand that in turn their beliefs are heavily influenced by what they have been taught or have inherited from their own upbringing and experiences. Their minds are likely to be full of fantasies about why you have PMS and what part they personally or men generally might have played in 'causing' it.

Sex is often still a taboo subject in this society and many of us grow up with the idea that sex is often the bringer of bad things. Sex education may teach us the 'nuts and bolts', but the rest is often covered in a rather confused mish-mash of moral precept and scare story. Men, as well as women, are frequently left with the feeling that the 'wages of sin' are sexual diseases, unwanted pregnancy and a broken heart. It is then a small step for a man to accept the false logic that if a woman is suffering from something like PMS it must be sex that has caused it. One step further and he can argue that since sex is something he sees as his doing to you then he must have caused whatever symptoms you are suffering. Any response he makes to the situation can then be coloured heavily by his feelings of guilt or his desire to avoid blame.

MALE MYTHS

To further understand why male responses to things sexual can seem somewhat off-target or even bizarre you have to consider some of the myths that influence them. Central to many of these are the very expressions we all learn very early in life to describe male sexual equipment. A large number of these expressions are violent – 'hard ons', 'horns', 'prick', 'dagger'. The language for sexual acts is equally aggressive – 'getting a leg over', 'poking', 'screwing', 'banging'. So it's hardly surprising that even very young men are soon confirmed in the idea that this mysterious thing called sex has the strength to hurt or do damage to women.

'My PMS got a lot worse around the time we'd been married about five years. Our relationship hit quite a rocky patch, and I would have said that it was the PMS getting bad that made me all uptight and that's what put a strain on our marriage. My husband says that things were going badly, and that's when I started getting tired and ratty just before my period. All I wanted was a bit of sympathy, but every time I said I was getting pains or felt bad he would just fly into a temper or work himself up into a slow burn that would go on for ages. He kept saying I was blaming him when I was doing nothing of the sort. I wanted to go to the doctor and get some treatment, and you would have thought that he would have been all for it, but he wasn't. In the end I had to go behind his back.'

This fear of the damaging potential of his own sexual power is what can be behind many men's unhelpful reactions to a partner having, talking about or seeking any form of treatment for her PMS. This reaction can be particularly strong if the PMS itself, or the treatment, in any way causes changes in your shared sexual activity or suggests that such changes should be made. If the man really does feel that he is at fault in what has happened, his own response can in some cases be as severe as his suffering impotence, in an unconscious attempt not to do you further harm. Or, he can go to the other extreme of having an affair, in another unconscious attempt to prove that he can have sex with another woman and do her no harm, and so prove he is blameless in the case where he has been 'accused'.

There is also a danger if you are aware of his having these sorts of fears that you can actually encourage them. This could be particularly so if you felt angry at his lack of sympathy or help, or if you and he already have any other areas of conflict. If, for example, sex between you has never really been all it might have been or has even become burdensome of late, being able to play on these fears could be seen to be a perfect way of lessening or even removing his sexual demands. You might be tempted to exaggerate your PMS symptoms or to pretend they continue to exist even though they had been removed or lessened by treatment.

WHAT ABOUT HIM?

As well as any worries he might have about what he may have done to you, your sexual partner is just as likely to have a pretty keen interest in what your condition and problems might be capable of doing to him. With PMS, as with any other 'illness', our most primitive beliefs can emerge. The strongest of these is fear of contamination. He might feel that what you have is somehow catching and that touching you, or even being with you, can in some way put him at risk. He can react in this manner even though every bit of his logic tells him that PMS cannot possibly be infectious. Sexual intercourse, probably our most intimate and complete example of touching, can become frightening rather than pleasurable. If PMS makes you depressed, in pain, physically clumsy or mentally slow, what on earth can contact with this monster be capable of doing to him? It is not surprising that sexual and other aspects of a relationship can become strained before, during and just after PMS symptoms emerge each month.

COMMUNICATION

If you are to deal successfully with your PMS and learn how to cope with it, ideally the men in your life – whether they are friends and colleagues, fathers and brothers, partners or sons – should help. It's a tall order to expect society at large to suddenly have a sea change, and for all of us to become aware and sympathetic about PMS. However, if we all started with the men who have close contact with us, this has to contribute to a wider change!

Communication is the first step. If you have a partner, involve him as fully as possible in the whole process of diagnosis or treatment, whether you are going the self-help, conventional medical or alternative therapy route. Any doctor or therapist you consult will respect your confidentiality above all and so may not even think to ask you if you want a partner involved at any stage. In one way this is understandable since it is ultimately your body and only you have the absolute right to say what will be done with it. However, since your PMS symptoms and their effects cannot be considered in isolation it makes common sense to ensure your partner is involved, even if you have to exert considerable persuasion to convince him of this. If he does resist your persuasion, you might be able to enlist the help of your GP, a district nurse or just a good friend to act as a go-between and help the two of you to get talking freely.

It will help if you can accept that very few men can recognise or acknowledge their fears in this area of their lives. Very few of them are able to overcome their embarrassment to ask the necessary questions, and the situation is not improved by the fact that very few men can pinpoint why the whole situation of women having problems in this way makes them feel so unsure and uneasy.

WORKING TOGETHER

PMS and any of its attendant problems is not an area where the old adage 'Least said, soonest mended' is going to be of any help to anyone. On the contrary, the more you and your partner, and indeed anyone else in your life, can talk openly, the more chance you will all have of dealing with the various aspects of your PMS. The process may be hard, but helping him to understand your fears and worries, and at the same time making it clear that you understand and can sympathise with his, can make all the difference. If you are lucky, all you will have to do is to bring it up as a subject for discussion and that will be that, the dialogue will be open and you will be on your way. However, it's more likely that you will be one of the majority of women who have some resistance that has to be overcome before their partner can be coaxed into involvement.

There are some well-tried techniques for opening the way to discussion, and if you are not getting immediate attention or co-operation from your man you could benefit from trying them.

'Betty has had funny days around her period ever since I've known her and it's not really a subject we much talked about. She left me this note saying that we needed to talk and I have to say I screwed it up and threw it away and did nothing. Then she left me a long letter about how she felt and what it did to her. It was quite an eye-opener and I came home all ready to talk and she had this magazine on the kitchen table, open at this article about PMS. I sat down and read it and said "That sounds just like the things you said in your letter." She said "Yes, that's just what it's like" and I asked her what she was going to do about it. She said "What do you suggest?" and we just went from there, really.'

It may seem unnaturally formal, or even at first faintly ridiculous, but writing a letter of explanation to him that he can read in his own time, in private, can be remarkably effective. So too can offering, or leaving to be found, books or magazines on the subject. There is something in the essential make-up of most men that makes information from a book or a magazine infinitely more acceptable to them than being talked to! All's fair in love and PMS and whether you inform him by mouth, letter or book, any way that enables him to understand and appreciate your problems and needs, and gives him an insight into his own reactions, can only help both of you. If he can be made aware of all of these things, especially if it can be done without him feeling he is the cause of them or needs to be guilty, you can change a helpless and sometimes antagonistic onlooker of a man into the ideal – an essential and supportive partner in your dealings with your PMS.

8

PMS and sex

PMS AND LACK OF DESIRE

How does PMS impact on your sex life? Sex and PMS tend to be seen as belonging to different categories, and are seldom talked about in the same breath. Medical problems are serious and sex is trivia, seems to be the idea. But, let's face it, lack of sexual desire is a common and major PMS symptom, and the way PMS can affect your sex life may be one of the main reasons for unhappiness and distress.

'I didn't go to my doctor for a long time because it was really embarrassing and anyway I didn't think he would take it seriously. I get PMS every month but I don't feel sick or anything or really get depressed. I just go off sex and don't feel like it at all. We both find it depressing. I hated it and I used to feel really guilty because I'd been making him miss out. I mean, the rest of the month would be fine but when I didn't feel like it I really didn't feel like it and it made both of us feel quite bad. But you don't feel doctors are there to help you have a good time in bed, do you?'

We know that most animals are only receptive to sexual arousal and may even only be able to have intercourse at certain times. They 'come into season' at particular, regular intervals. In contrast, human females are receptive or potentially able to have sex at any time in the month, any time of the year. But being able to perform the act or even being able to become aroused is not exactly the same thing as being continuously sexually responsive. Perhaps PMS is part of a mechanism that is a left-over from our seasonal ancestors. Throughout a menstrual cycle, there are particular times when we are more, or less, responsive. There may be a very good reason for these variations in feeling. Just as the uncomfortable sensation of PMS may be an evolutionary 'rap on the knuckles' for not getting pregnant, so there may be a 'carrot and stick' effect in the way we do or do not feel like making love at certain points.

Generally speaking, you may find yourself particularly keen on having sex mid-way between periods. This coincides with ovulation, when you are most likely to get pregnant. You may find yourself least keen just before your period – when you have 'failed' in your biological purpose and not fallen pregnant. Nature wants you to save your efforts for a week or so, until you could have another go at perpetuating the species and so pours cold water on the whole business of having a good time in bed that night!

All women are individuals, and not all experience these monthly fluctuations, or only do so to a mild degree. Being on the Pill or breastfeeding can also flatten out any periodic swings in sexual feelings, or libido, and produce a less erratic sexual response. Given the right partner, the right mood and the right setting, any woman may be happy to be sexually aroused, whatever her rhythm or hormones are telling her. So, neither PMS nor monthly rhythms can be made an absolute scapegoat for any sexual relationship that doesn't gel. But if we accept the fact that some three-quarters of women do have a degree of PMS and that the majority do react to monthly hormonal changes, then we should be able to recognise our own pattern, and share this information with our sexual partners. That way, a good sexual relationship could follow the ups and downs of desire and sensation through the monthly cycle, taking advantage of the times when intense stimulation would be welcome or when only the lightest touch would be needed. This would also allow both of you to know when sex would be best left out of the night's activities and you'd rather opt for a cuddle, without either of you feeling hurt or rejected.

Many factors combine to make any one of us in the mood for love at any particular moment. The most obvious stimulus, of course, is the right partner! But your general mood contributes to your chances of ending up in bed. If you've had a tiring day at work or at home, you may not feel up to it. But, in fact, your energy levels may be less important than your sense of self-esteem and confidence arising from the day's events. In short, if you've had a tiring but successful day you may well be feeling amorous, while a restful but disappointing day may leave you feeling deflated.

But physical rhythms may also play a part in your sexual readiness, or lack of it. The rise and fall of hormones during your menstrual cycle not only ready your reproductive organs for pregnancy; they also ready the rest of you for sex. Most women will find that their sexual feelings will be at a peak just before ovulation, falling afterwards, with a slight raise in the premenstruum. They may find they experience increased sensitivity to touch before and during the period of ovulation, with less responsiveness after and in the premenstruum, rising again during their period. So you could say that it would be 'natural' for any woman to have times in the month when she would be more or less keen to have sex and that the type of sex she welcomes may also change from day to day. At times of increased sensitivity, when hormonal changes have filled tissues with extra fluid, she may be particularly eager for hot and heavy sex. On days when breasts are tender and lumpy, she may prefer sex to be slow and gentle. In the main, it would seem that sex is especially welcome at two points in the menstrual cycle; when she is most likely to get pregnant, around ovulation, and when she is least likely, during her period. It's almost as if nature designed us to have 'businesstime sex' for the continuation of the species and 'playtime sex' for fun!

This would be the pattern for the women without PMS problems, but if we overlay this with the symptoms of severe or mild PMS, there can be further and often dramatic changes. Severe sufferers come off worst, particularly in the few days before a period starts which, without their symptoms, may normally be a time of increased sexual arousal. Far from being aroused and receptive, the severe sufferer finds that her sex urges can be extremely reduced. Frequently she does not even want to be touched, let alone have intercourse. It is more likely to be a time of headaches, irritation and arguments, and if she is pushed into having sex by an insensitive partner, it will often be painful and unpleasant. Symptoms such as tender breasts, a swollen abdomen and an inability to relax will combine to make lovemaking unattractive to her at this time.

MILD PMS AND INCREASED SENSITIVITY

The woman who has mild PMS is almost the opposite of her severely stricken sister. Her sensitivity increases, especially her breasts, and she reacts to the lightest caress and she may feel a greater need for orgasmic release. One explanation offered for this need for orgasm is that premenstrual fluid retention in the tissues causes a heightened physical awareness of the labia minora and the clitoris.

Some women also report an enhanced deep vaginal sensitivity at this time.

Mild PMS can turn you into a wonderwoman on speed, showing sudden and sometimes uncharacteristic bursts of energy and activity – spring cleaning the house, cooking enough food for an army, shopping for the week, doing two gym classes and still at the end of a busy day having enough energy left to be calling out for sex. However, if good sex is to be enjoyed when you have mild PMS, it will only be if your partner is aware of your greater physical tenderness at this time and you both adjust your sexual techniques accordingly. Tender, gentle sex is going to get the best results for both of you. Extreme sensitivity to any form of physical stimulation means it will be a real case of softly softly catchee sexy monkey. A too-heavy hand will quickly turn a delightful caress into an unwelcome irritation, and any over-enthusiastic hand on a bloated breast or thrusting into a hair-triggered vagina is going to give pain rather than pleasure.

The most common response that appears in questionnaires to women with mild PMS is that, while they experience increased arousal, they usually like to take things gently. It might help a man to understand a woman's responses at this time if he tries to think of her state in his terms. Most men would accept that if they wanted to get the release that an orgasm would bring, they would rather stroke themselves slowly and gently with a smooth, oiled hand than give themselves a damned good seeing to with a handy piece of sandpaper. Both methods would probably get you there in the end, but going the rough and ready sandpaper route would leave all but the most dedicated masochist feeling somewhat disenchanted with the whole experience.

PMS and a sex life is not all abstinence, major adjustments, dire warnings or doom and gloom on the bedroom front at this time of the month. Some women find their increased physical sensitivity at PMS time is combined with feelings of dreaminess and lethargy. Instead of spending the premenstruum bouncing off walls in frenetic activities they feel sensual, luxurious and laid back. Given the choice, you may want to spend most of the time lazing in bed with your favourite goodies or your favourite man. It can be a marvellous few days of slow and lazy lovemaking when you could both reach very sexy heights that you might not climb on other days in the month. Again, you will only get there if the man is aware and is sensitive, considerate and tender.

BEYOND PENETRATIVE SEX

One very important aspect to consider is that lovemaking does not need to be penetrative to be satisfying. Trying to make a case for heterosexual non-penetrative sex is not easy. We seem to find it almost impossible to adjust our thinking that the only *real* sex is penis in vagina and that anything else is either a poor imitation or a 'failure'.

Too many of us still seem to see intercourse as the only purpose of sexual contact. This produces intercourse-centred or target sex, which has limitations. Penetrative sex is not necessarily the most intimate thing a couple can do together. If you can look beyond the mystic significance that is attached to virginity and penetration you can realise that intercourse is actually *less* intimate, and less satisfying, than many other sexual acts between two people. This is probably exactly why so many of us, in adolescence, skip straight to 'going the whole way', and miss out on 'petting'. After all, it was often actually easier to have or allow intercourse than to negotiate, give or receive other physical intimacies.

Some indication of how sex is seen by large numbers of people and why penetration persists as the *only* way is the language, and the gender of that language, we use to describe it. The Inuit have over 20 words for 'snow' and when you live surrounded by the stuff for most of your life this bid for a little bit of variety could be said to be reasonable, but our own multiplicity of words for sex seems to be driven by needs stronger and often darker than mere variety. There is a heavy presence of words that suggest power, competition, dominance and separateness between the sexes, and the need for speed in the sexual act. There are very few slang words for love, intimacy or the desire to linger in or extend sexual contact.

An obsession with penetrative sex may come about, not because men are in a hurry for some ultimate pleasure, but because their fear of being swallowed or bitten by the vagina makes them want to get it over with as quickly as possible. Sadly, if PMS is a factor, the link between sex and pain or bad moods may make this fear even greater. And when women say that lack of sexual desire may be one of their PMS symptoms, what may be happening is that they have no desire for *sexual intercourse* at this time. They would still, often, very much welcome either gentle and sensual comfort, or indeed touching to orgasm.

'I'm simply turned off sex in the week or so before my period. I feel very bloated and my breasts get tender, and I just can't bear to be grabbed – it sets my teeth on edge. My partner and I used to have a bad time because it seemed he always wanted sex at this time and I was always pushing him away, and we'd end up in screaming rows. He came back one day and said he'd figured it out. What he didn't like was that I turned away from him and it made him feel I didn't love him or want *him*, not just sex. I like being held and I love having a back rub at this time, but I'd avoid asking for it because I thought he'd think I wanted sex and try it on, and then I'd just push him off and we'd be in a row again. So we cuddle and sometimes I'll say "Give us a back rub" and he'll say "Well, give us a rub too"! And I'll use my hands on him, and that suits both of us. And sometimes I feel like it too, and coming makes me feel relaxed. It's the full thing – penetration – that I don't like at this time. Mind you, it's made sex at other times of the month even better now, because we know how to take a bit of time at it and how to do other things that get us going.'

SEX AND PERIODS

If a loss of sexual desire during the premenstruum is one of your symptoms, that may at least mean your sexual feelings come back again as soon as your period begins. You and your partner, however, may experience a problem with this.

'Since my PMS has got worse, we only make love a couple of times a month, if we're lucky. I do miss it, specially those months when we've got a lot on the go and some nights when we could get together, we're both too tired. There's about a week to ten days after my period when I feel great, and then I get bad and then, of course, it's my period when you can't do anything.'

It would seem logical, that as soon as the effects of PMS have faded, you might like to take advantage of the upswing in your mood. But is this always so? The fact is that sex and periods are another of society's taboos.

Rationally speaking, one form of body fluid is much the same as any other. If you don't find vaginal lubrication or semen dirty or unpleasant, why should you find period blood any more so? Many people do, and feelings of distaste or even fear of menstruation, and particularly disgust at the thought of having sex during a period, are not new. The Bible tells us that a menstruating woman, and everyone and everything that touches her 'shall be unclean'. The Roman naturalist Pliny then added his own horrors when he wrote that contact with menstrual blood, 'Turns new wines sour, crops touched by it become barren, grafts die, seeding gardens are dried up, the fruit of trees fall off, the edge of steel and the gleam of ivory are dulled, hives of bees die, even bronze and iron are at once seized by rust and a horrible smell fills the air: to taste it drives dogs mad and infects their bites with an incurable poison.' These may be old views, but blood, and particularly menstrual blood, still has powerful associations for many people.

This is a pity, since sex during the time that a woman has her period can have positive benefits. Some women find lovemaking to orgasm a particular bonus during a period, as the action of arousal and orgasm can relieve the discomfort of period pains. Both men and women can be excited by the sense of breaking a taboo; 'naughty, messy' sex can be seen as especially arousing. Orgasms can be different during menstruation. Although some women find their sensations are no different from other times of the month, others discover they are quicker to orgasm, while some experience slower, deeper climaxes. What periods certainly don't do is stop you from being satisfied. Sex at this time of the month has a particular facet for PMS sufferers, because the difficulties you may be having with your PMS may have compressed the time during the month when you feel like having sex. The drawback of that may be that your PMS can make you feel sad and lacking in self-esteem; losing out on the intimate side of your relationship can do the same, so you suffer a double dose of misery. If, as is very common, the only reason you do not take advantage of the lifting of PMS symptoms to enjoy your sex life is that you think having sex at this time is wrong, you would be missing out.

Pregnancy and periods

Sex during a period can also have an extra edge if you usually use a method of contraception that you feel is less efficient than you would like. Fears of pregnancy may make you slightly apprehensive at most other times, but these anxieties can be absent during a period. While some people like, or indeed need, that extra edge to spice up their sex lives, for most people a fear of pregnancy acts as a brake on their sexual urges, preventing them from truly letting go and enjoying their lovemaking to the full.

However, if you do decide to overcome any previous inhibitions and have sex at the time of your period, do not take chances and ignore the fact that you can still put yourself at the risk of pregnancy at this time. If you have a short cycle – say, only two weeks between the end of one period and the beginning of another – you may ovulate very quickly after the first day of your period. Sperm may be able to survive in the fallopian tubes for up to five days after ejaculation. If you make love during a period in the mistaken belief that your flow of menstrual blood will get rid of the semen, you could in fact be made pregnant when at ovulation an egg emerges to find still viable sperm waiting in the fallopian tube. In spite of the flow of blood, active, vigorous sperm will still be able to swim up from the vagina through the uterus and into the fallopian tubes during your period. A sticky fluid is produced by the cervix and forms a fairly effective barrier to sperm in the days after and before your period. It turns to a welcoming passageway for sperm during ovulation when your body wishes to encourage a possibility of conception. This sticky barrier is also absent during menstruation, and the flow of menstrual blood does not perform the same function. So it's always wise to use precautions even then. If you are on the Pill, however, protection extends throughout the month, as long as you are taking it correctly.

The reduction in vaginal lubrication during menstruation does create a problem other than that of lack of contraceptive protection. Sex during menstruation can seem dry and uncomfortable, if not painful. Furthermore, if you want to do something to hold back the flow while you make love, you may find the vagina even drier and more uncomfortable. For this reason additional lubrication may be particularly important at this time. You can use lubricating gels such as KY or Durex lubricating jelly which you will find on open sale at your pharmacy. You can also use spermicidal jelly which would have the additional advantage, if you were using a barrier method for contraceptive or protective purposes, of containing nonoxynol-9 which kills both sperm and many organisms that lead to sexual infections.

Sexual infection is the only danger that can be associated with having sex during a period. Period blood itself is sterile until it is exposed to air and begins to decay, so it cannot harm your partner and neither can his semen harm you at this time. However, if either of you has a sexual infection, both partners would be more vulnerable to contracting it or passing it on if you are having sex during a period. So, if you are normally using the safer sex techniques to prevent your partner's body fluids coming into contact with your bloodstream, such as using a male or female condom or not having penetrative sex, go on using these precautions even during a period.

How to

If you and your partner would like to have sex during menstruation but aren't happy about the actual mechanics of it, there are various ways in which you can make sure that neither you nor your bed get too messy in the process. You can contain the flow in a number of ways. You can insert a contraceptive diaphragm or a contraceptive sponge. If you are using these for contraceptive purposes, leave them in place for the recommended six hours after you have made love. If you don't need to use these for birth control, you can take them out as soon as you like. If contraception is not an issue, you could also use a small piece of natural sponge. These can be used instead of tampons and as long as they are kept clean they are not a health risk. Making love with a tampon in place is not, however, recommended. They are less flexible than sponges and can cause pain, or become wedged behind the pubic bone and difficult to remove without help. Keeping back the flow of your period by using a cap is not a health risk, although you should never leave anything in the vagina for too long. Tampons and sponges should generally be removed and changed during menstruation at least every 3 to 4 hours, and the maximum time you are recommended to leave a sponge or diaphragm in place for contraceptive purposes is 30 hours.

Choices

Plenty of couples avoid sex for the duration of a period, but many of them never get round to discussing whether this is to both their tastes. When talking about a subject as difficult as this, it's often useful to have some trigger material to spark off a discussion. A magazine article, or a chapter such as this is ideal, and you could use it to show to your partner and say 'What do you think about this?'

Sex *is* a squishy, messy business at the best of times and that is often what is such fun about it. Little girls and boys enjoy messing around in puddles, squeezing mud between their toes and building channels in the sand, for the sheer sensual delight of it. It's a moot point whether sex is such fun because it reminds you of those pleasures, or both pleasures spring from the same well. Some people carry these delights a stage further and enhance lovemaking with creams and oils. Whatever, the chances are that your instinctive feelings about sex during a period will be more inclined to seeing it as a pleasure rather than recoiling in disgust.

It's only an inherited social convention that has made the idea of having sex during a woman's period less than appealing, and it's up to you whether you wish to retain that conditioned attitude or not. What is absolutely certain is that you don't *have* to have sex at this time of the month if you don't want to. In fact, you don't have to have sex at any time in the month if you're not feeling like it. This isn't being prudish. It's all a matter of choice and, as always, you have the right to make your own choices. But you certainly don't have to deny yourself if this is something you would like to do, and both you and your partner might find it a source of considerable pleasure and comfort at what could otherwise be a stressful time.

9

What can be done with conventional therapy

We have already seen that there is enormous disagreement about definitions and descriptions of PMS. When it comes to looking at treatments there is even more confusion. You may not be surprised to learn that in a recent survey over half of the doctors in Britain questioned admitted that they experienced some difficulty in treating PMS.

> 'When I saw my doctor the first time, she didn't say anything you could put your finger on, but I felt she was quite off with me. She told me later that it was because she hates it when people come in with PMS because she feels she's on a loser from the start. I was lucky because what she tried with me worked and I've been much better since I went, although it took a few months for it to come through properly. But she says she has some women whom she's been seeing for years and nothing seems to make the slightest bit of difference, or it works for a time and then they are back to square one.'

The main problem is that scientific studies constantly and consistently disagree with word-of-mouth evidence about which treatments are effective. There are many enthusiastic followers of various PMS treatments, from vitamin supplements to diets to hormonal treatments. These treatments are all dogged with the same problem. This is that when you compare them in a properly conducted trial, any inactive therapy (termed a placebo), designed to allow you to compare what will happen when a woman is given the therapy as opposed to when she is given something else, is likely to show just as good a result. Some 50 per cent of women appear to initially respond to placebo treatment and some doctors see this as confirming the old belief that PMS is 'all in the mind'. The more general, modern opinion is that this simply underlines the complexity of the mixture of the emotional or hormonal causes of PMS.

This mixture or interrelation of the causes of PMS is understandable if you recognise that the hormones which drive the menstrual cycle are produced (or their production is triggered) by a part of the brain, the hypothalamus, and the small gland at the base of the brain, the pituitary. The hypothalamus is extremely responsive to emotional states, and stress or ill-health will affect hormonal output. Just as there is no clear-cut single cause of PMS, so there is often no single or absolute cure for its symptom or symptoms. A final complication is added by our attitudes to some of the possible treatments that are on offer. Many people, for example, are unhappy with conventional medicine, particularly with the use of artificial hormones. An increasing number of people are opting for one of the other main methods of treatment: psychotherapy, non-hormone drug therapy, nutrition supplements and a change of eating habits. Using natural or alternative medicine will be examined fully in Chapter 10.

In spite of the apparent wealth of 'cures' on offer, your best route is to try whatever you or your doctor, or other sources, think may help you among the various options and then persist until you find the one or the combination that is best for you.

YOU AND YOUR DOCTOR

Whatever treatment is going to be considered or given to you, you will get the best results if you can achieve real communication with your doctor or any other of your advisers. The professional experts may have the skills to diagnose what is wrong and what could be done, but you have the final word. You can't take this decision unless you have the most complete picture possible of what is happening to your body and what needs to be done about it. It makes sense, therefore, that you take in as much information as possible each time you visit your doctor or other adviser. This may not be easy if, like so many of us visiting a doctor, you find your mind goes blank or goes into 'intermittent mode' during the consultation. It's then that you find yourself coming away clutching a prescription you don't understand or emerge with your ears ringing with the doctor's reassurance but somehow don't feel at all reassured. This is not going to help you with something as potentially complicated as PMS, so try the following strategies for successful surgery visits.

Make a list of all the questions you want answered and take this list with you. Some of the questions you may want answered to your full satisfaction could be among the following.

- Do I have PMS?
- Can you find any medical reasons for my symptoms?
- If I don't have PMS, what other causes could there be for my symptoms?
- How can you help me?
- What are the full details of any medicines or treatments you suggest?
- How will any medicines work and what side effects could there be?

- What can I do for myself?
- Where do I go from here?

Add you own to this list! Make sure they are *all* answered to your satisfaction. If you think you would be taking up too much time in a routine appointment, ask for one that will allow the doctor a longer time to deal with you fully. If you are not happy with the way your doctor deals with you, or this particular situation, do say so. We tend to shy away from questioning or confronting doctors. We often feel that a doctor is doing us a favour in seeing us. Because money does not change hands, we often think we are being seen out of charity and the goodness of the doctor's heart. Not so! Doctors are paid, out of our contributions, so we have as much right to expect good care as if the payment were direct. We also seem to think they are always in the right, and always know what they are doing. But they are human, too. As already suggested, one reason for apparent lack of sympathy could be that they feel at a loss while all their training says that they *should* have an answer. Pointing out that they are being less than helpful *may* get you 'a flea in the ear'! But it may enable the doctor to share his or her own sense of frustration and helplessness.

You can always ask for a second opinion, as well. You have the right, while remaining with your present doctor, to ask another one for his or her views on the condition you are wanting investigating. The only drawback is that while you have the right to ask this, and your doctor should agree, your doctor is the person who chooses whom you see for this. And they can, if they choose, just send you to another doctor in their own practice. However, while another doctor in the same practice may hold the same opinions as your doctor's, they may not, so it is always worth going along if this is offered. If your doctor remains totally unhelpful, don't forget that you can switch doctors to a more helpful one. You simply take your medical card to a new doctor and ask to be taken on their list. You can ask for an interview with them first, to find out their attitudes and see if you will get on.

'My GP was a total dead loss when it had to do with sex or periods. I'd tried to get help for years and then a friend who signed on with a younger doctor in the same practice said that I should see her as she was really good. I didn't know you could change doctors, not without a good reason that is, and I didn't realise that you didn't have to give a reason but just ask to be taken on. So I moved to the new doctor and when I did see her I felt much better about talking to her because she listened.'

So, what treatments *can* your doctor offer you?

HORMONES

If we are to accept the theory that PMS is caused by an upset or an imbalance in hormone levels associated with the menstrual cycle it would follow that PMS may be treated by giving natural or artificial hormones to restore a normal balance. Treatment that interferes with ovulation and produces a change in your cycle – such as progesterone, oestrogen, oestrogen and progestogen, danazol and GnRH analogues – are most successful with PMS symptoms such as cramps, abdominal pains or bloating.

Progesterone/Progestogen

Progesterone has been targeted by the doctor who put PMS on the map, Dr Katharina Dalton, as being at the centre of the PMS problem. If PMS is a condition that occurs because the body is not getting enough progesterone or is having some difficulty dealing with the progesterone that is naturally present, it would stand to reason that treatment with this hormone should put things right. Progesterone is often therefore offered either as progesterone, which is a naturally occurring form, or as progestogen, which is the synthetic version.

There are two problems with using progesterone. The first is that progesterone is difficult to produce to be taken by mouth as tablets. It is usually given as injections, or by implants. It can also be given through suppositories, which are inserted in the back passage, or pessaries which are inserted in the vagina. The other drawback is that progesterone was originally made from animal sources. While some is now extracted from vegetable sources, some is still made in the original way. If you are an animal lover, being offered a treatment which may involve cruelty to animals can certainly put you off it. However, progesterone *is* now produced from vegetable sources, involving no cruelty. If this is an issue with you, ask your doctor to check out the origin of any progesterone prescribed to you.

The problem as stated by doctors in favour of using progesterone as a PMS treatment is that progestogen, the synthetic form, is ineffective, or not as effective as progesterone. However, there is very little reliable research to show that either progesterone or progestogen are outstanding treatments for PMS. Dalton has treated thousands of women with progesterone and is enthusiastic about the results. I'm not aware, however, that she has conducted any controlled studies into this treatment. I believe her view is that, since the positive evidence is so overwhelming, it would be wrong to deny any sufferers this therapy by making them controls in a study.

Micronised oral progesterone was used in one controlled study and produced significant results in reducing anxiety, depression, stress, swelling, fluid retention and hot flushes, but not in loss of sexual interest or restlessness. Unfortunately it was also associated with severe premenstrual headaches. Two researchers, Maxson and Hargrove, noted drowsiness and dizziness in as many as one-third of cycles treated.

However, the many controlled studies on progesterone that have been done by other researchers do not confirm the claim that it is the answer. At best, claims for progesterone still need to be substantiated. As in so much PMS therapy, placebo pills often seem to give as good a result. Theoretically progesterone can relieve bloating, period pains, and the nausea, vomiting and diarrhoea often associated with PMS. Since it functions as a muscle relaxant and sedative, it may be prescribed for PMS, stress or tension.

Since many people report success with progesterone and progestogen, as with many PMS treatments it is well worth trying. If it doesn't work for you, don't despair. The danger of being told that one particular treatment is the magic solution is that, if it doesn't work for you, you may feel that you have done something wrong or that you are particularly unusual. You haven't, and you aren't, and the answer would be to simply go on looking for a solution.

Progesterone and progestogen are only available on a doctor's prescription. They are usually given from mid-cycle to the onset of menstruation. If progesterone is going to have an effect, unlike many treatments it is likely to be noticeable in the first or second cycle of treatment.

Oestrogen

It has been suggested that PMS could be treated by altering ovulation, with oestrogen given as an implant or a skin patch. The problem with using oestrogen in this way is that, over a course of time, oestrogen on its own has harmful effects on the lining of the womb. You would have to give progestogen as well to protect the lining. As with most PMS studies, the results of using oestrogen have been confusing and inconclusive. Oestrogen is only available on a doctor's prescription.

Oestrogen and Progestogen

If you want to block ovulation one obvious way of doing it would be to use the oral contraceptive pill. After all, that is the whole point of this particular preparation. In early studies of the Pill some women said that when using it their PMS symptoms improved. However, some of the women in these studies also said that their PMS symptoms worsened. These studies were not looking at PMS but at the contraceptive effectiveness of the Pill and the evidence about PMS was gathered from women remarking on how they thought the Pill had or had not affected them. Therefore, they can't really be said to give an accurate picture. Later studies have given a confused picture suggesting that some symptoms such as breast pain and period-type pain may be better on the combined pills but that mood changes may be worse.

One advantage of the oral contraceptive is that you can manipulate its use not only to eliminate ovulation but periods as well. If you are on the form of combined oral contraceptive that delivers the same formula of hormones throughout the month, you may simply go from one packet straight on to another without having a pill-free break. It's perfectly safe to do this and quite a few women regularly take four packets one after the other, so having a period every three months rather than monthly. As with many other treatments, results vary from person to person and there is no conclusive evidence one way or the other. You may like to try this for yourself, having talked it over with your doctor. At the moment the oral contraceptive pill is only available on a doctor's prescription.

Danazol

As we have already seen, one theory on the cause of PMS is an imbalance in the progestogen to oestrogen ratio during a particular phase of the menstrual cycle. PMS is not present before you start your periods and disappears after you finish them at menopause. It also tends not to be present in women who have had their ovaries removed. So a possible treatment is stop ovarian activity through drug treatment. Danazol (brand name Danol) is a drug that does this. It is a synthetic form of the male hormone testosterone. Danazol has an anti-gonadotrophin effect. This means that it interferes with the pituitary's production of two hormones, FSH and LH. Because the surge of these hormones is reduced and oestrogen production is discouraged, periods and ovulation will stop.

There have been reports that danazol is effective in dealing with breast pain, anxiety, tiredness and food cravings, but that it is less effective with other PMS symptoms. However, to prevent ovulation and periods a fairly high dose needs to be given and side effects are then fairly common, which is why danazol tends only to be suggested if other treatments have been unsuccessful. Since danazol has the effect of making the body more masculine, body hair can increase while head hair becomes thinner. Weight gain and acne are fairly common, as are depression, tiredness and joint pains. Some women also find their voice deepens. At lesser doses, danazol has been reported as relieving some symptoms without either blocking ovulation or altering menstrual bleeding. The theory is that it does so through a range of complex effects which make it difficult for it to be prescribed with consistent results. It is only available on prescription from your doctor.

GnRH

There are other ways of blocking ovulation. One is by using gonadotrophin-releasing hormone (GnRH), also called luteinising-hormone-releasing hormone (LHRH), analogues. These are synthetic substances that act on the pituitary gland. They act like the chemicals that tell your pituitary to produce the hormones that trigger oestrogen production. GnRH analogues can either be antagonists or agonists. An antagonist works by discouraging the pituitary from producing its hormones. An agonist works by stimulating the pituitary, prompting it to produce hormones all the time instead of in pulses as it normally would. The result with an agonist is the same in the end as using an antagonist, because the pituitary reacts to being told to work full time by switching itself off or 'down regulating'. GnRH agonists can be prescribed as a nasal spray, as implants in a slow-release capsule inserted under the skin, or taken by mouth. Side effects can be the sort of reactions you might expect at menopause, such as hot flushes, vaginal dryness, night sweats, loss of sexual feelings, breast tenderness, tiredness and irritability. As with all hormone therapy, they are only available on a doctor's prescription.

SURGERY

If stopping ovulation is the cure for PMS, then the most drastic and complete way to do that would be to surgically remove the ovaries altogether. This is a treatment that is sometimes suggested in intractable cases of PMS. It is, however, a step from which you cannot return and all the implications of it should be seriously considered before any decision to go this route is taken. If you remove the ovaries it is also wise to remove the womb, since otherwise you may be encouraging future problems with the endometrium, the lining of the womb. Removal of both ovaries, a bi-lateral oophorectomy, would only be suggested in a woman who had completed her family and is at the age when she would be nearing natural menopause. This is because, if you have your ovaries removed and do not then take oestrogen as a hormone replacement therapy (HRT), you are increasing your risks of suffering the dangerous, bone-thinning condition of osteoporosis. A catch-22 can then emerge since, if you take artificial oestrogen as HRT, there is always the risk that you may experience your PMS symptoms again. If you have your ovaries removed and cannot take HRT, there are treatments and supplements you can take to deal with the increased risk of osteoporosis.

If surgery is considered, you are advised to test out whether removal of your ovaries may work for you by experiencing a so-called 'medical oophorectomy', by taking either danazol or a GnRH analogue for a time. If you didn't get any relief it would call into question whether removing your ovaries would actually give you any benefit. After a trial three months, you and your doctor might like to consider your options.

NON-HORMONE DRUG THERAPY

Bromocriptine

Bromocriptine (brand name Parlodel) is used for conditions due to the over-production in the body of prolactin. This hormone stimulates breast tissue, which is why bromocriptine, which inhibits secretion of prolactin from the pituitary gland, may be prescribed when the complaint is of breast pain or tenderness. An increase in prolactin might also account for psychological symptoms. In one study, women with increased prolactin reported more symptoms of depression than did the control subjects and these were reduced when treated with bromocriptine.

Bromocriptine is given as tablets or capsules. Side effects are usually dose-related, which means that the higher the dose the more likely you are to get them. Dizziness is fairly common, and so too are nausea and vomiting, although these can be reduced if you take your tablets with meals.

However, side effects mean that bromocriptine is unlikely to be offered as a long-term solution, and is only available on prescription from your doctor.

Interestingly, at least two studies have pointed out that prolactin is secreted during sleep and investigated the result of sleep deprivation. Staying awake may be a novel way of treating PMS, but according to these studies it worked for a significant number of sufferers.

Anti-anxiety and anti-depressant drugs

If depression or anxiety are part of or the main symptoms in your PMS, you may find that drugs to tackle these states directly are offered to you. Messages are passed around both your brain and your body by chemicals. You would obviously want to feel alert and on edge if you needed to react to an emergency. Anxiety, however, can be the unpleasant result if you keep having feelings of nervousness and tension with no obvious source and which you have no way of dealing with. Usually anxiety is best dealt with by counselling or psychotherapy to find out why it is happening and then dealing with the cause rather than just with the symptoms. However, anxiety can be dealt with directly by using drugs that attach themselves to brain cells and block the action of the 'anxiety' chemicals. Anxiety as a symptom of PMS may be dealt with in this way. The two main classes of drugs used to deal with anxiety are the benzodiazepines, such as Diazepam and Lorazepam, and the beta blockers such as Propranolol. Benzodiazepines tend to deal with the emotional results, acting on the fear and unhappiness felt. Beta blockers act on the physical symptoms of anxiety such as shaking, breathlessness and palpitations.

Anti-depressants are used to treat depression. There are two main types, tricyclic anti-depressants and monoamine oxidase inhibitors (MAOIs). All anti-depressants work by increasing the levels of certain chemicals in your brain called neurotransmitters. When brain chemistry is normal, neurotransmitters are constantly being released, and then reabsorbed and broken down. Their effect is to stimulate your moods. When you are depressed, fewer neuro-transmitters are released. Your brain cells reabsorb them but, since there are fewer, the cells are not as stimulated as they would normally be.

Tricyclic anti-depressants prevent brain cells reabsorbing the neurotransmitters so that they float around in the brain continuing to be stimulating for longer. MAOIs inhibit the enzyme that normally breaks down the neurotransmitters, so again these build up in the brain and continue to stimu-late. Tricyclic anti-depressants may take from at least 10 to 14 days to begin to have a beneficial effect and may take even longer. However, their side effects can make them-selves felt very quickly. Common side effects with tricyc-lics are dry mouth, difficulty in passing water, drowsiness, dizziness, blurred vision and constipation.

If you are using MAOIs you have to avoid anything which has tyramine in it. This includes cheese, Marmite or any other yeast extract, meat extracts, alcohol, especially red wine, and chocolate. This is because mixing MAOIs and tyramine could result in a dangerous increase in blood pressure. All treatment with either anti-anxiety or anti-depressant drugs is by a doctor's prescription only. The dosages of these drugs and the duration of any course of treatment will depend on the severity of the symptoms you are experiencing.

Anti-prostaglandin drugs

Prostaglandins are substances that are released from cells in your body when the cells are damaged in any way. Pros-taglandins have the effect of stimulating pain – their job, in effect, is to draw the body's attention to the fact that something is wrong. That sort of warning is useful if you can then go ahead and do something about it. What should happen, of course, is that your body systems themselves react and correct whatever is wrong. But, if you are suffering chronic pain because your body can't deal with what is happening and medical science either can't diagnose the problem or can diagnose it but can't treat it properly, then the warning signal becomes redundant and intolerable. In which case, your main interest at this point would be the relief of any pain.

There are various drugs that block the production of prostaglandins such as aspirin, paracetamol and ibuprofen. The most effective in treating PMS-related pains, as well as general period pains, is mefenamic acid (brand name Ponstan). The side effects of using this may include indigestion or diarrhoea and, like any other painkiller, Ponstan shouldn't be taken over a prolonged period or mixed with alcohol. The anti-prostaglandin drugs are most effective in treating the pains of PMS if they are taken one or two days before symptoms usually start and for a further couple of days after the onset of a period.

Some women find that preparations that combine codeine with one of the anti-prostaglandin drugs are even more effective. Most of these painkillers are available over-the-counter and dosages will be stated on their packets. It is advisable to respect and pay strict attention to these since most popular painkillers can have damaging effects if taken in too large a quantity. If you have any digestive or liver problems or asthma you should take particular care. Mefenamic acid is obtainable on prescription only.

Diuretics

Diuretics help to turn excess fluid in the body into urine. This means you increase the number of times you go to the loo and the amount of water you pass. They may be prescribed if bloating and cyclical weight gain due to fluid retention is one of your problems. What happens normally is that as blood passes through your kidneys, waste products are filtered out, along with water, sodium and potassium salts. Most of the water and the salts go back into the bloodstream, while the waste products, some of the salts and some of the water are passed out of the body as urine. Diuretics have a blocking action, so instead of being reabsorbed, the sodium plus water and potassium are passed out instead. The drawbacks with diuretics are that they make you thirsty, and once you stop using them there can be a 'rebound' effect and you can retain even more fluid.

There are several different groups of diuretics. With some you can lose a lot of potassium and with others you can have the opposite effect of retaining too much potassium. Side effects of nausea and dizziness are not uncommon. Products which offer a diuretic action are also available over the counter without prescription. These usually contain caffeine which certainly makes you pass water, but can also have a highly stimulating effect. Not only can this keep you awake but it can increase any anxiety you may be having at an already stressful time. Diuretics are usually taken as tablets once daily while you are having active symptoms, usually at breakfast. They are generally only prescribed for short-time use for PMS.

Some interesting research suggests that not only is premenstrual bloating a normal aspect of cyclical change but that it isn't associated with an actual increase in girth. Fluid may shift around in your body and there may be an increase in distension or pressure in your gut, making you feel stretched and tight, but your actual external measurements don't increase. The feeling of bloatedness is enough to make clothing uncomfortable and waistbands feel too snug – enough to make you feel acutely uncomfortable and in need of clothes a size larger than those you usually use.

But on an objective measurement, your size hasn't actually increased. If this is so, diuretics would not be an appropriate treatment.

NUTRITIONAL SUPPLEMENTS

Vitamins are complex chemicals which are essential to a healthy body. There are 13 major vitamins – A, C, D, E, K and 8 B complex vitamins. Minerals are elements such as calcium, sodium or selenium that are found, often in tiny amounts, in food and are essential to a healthy working of the body. It has been suggested that vitamin and mineral deficiencies may be associated with PMS, and certainly some women do find that vitamin and mineral supplements can help with their symptoms. It must be stressed, however, that supplements should never be seen as replacing a healthy diet. If you are going to use them you should look to your eating patterns at the same time, and see the supplements as aiding and abetting good eating rather than being an alternative.

Vitamin B6 (pyridoxine)

Pyridoxine (B6) works to assist the healthy functioning of your brain and nervous system, your digestion, your skin, muscles, blood and metabolism. You need at least 2 mg of pyridoxine every day in a healthy diet, and the vitamin can be found occurring naturally in red and white meat, liver, eggs, fish, cereals and bread. It is particularly found in white meat such as chicken, oily fish such as mackerel, liver and in whole-grain cereal. Pyridoxine is also found in bananas, avocados and potatoes.

Being on the Pill is said to increase your B6 requirement. A vegetarian, and especially a vegan, diet can be deficient in this vitamin. One hundred grams of pulses and vegetables may only contain 0.16 mg, and 100 g of whole-meal bread only 0.14 mg, while 100 g of mackerel or liver would contain 0.7 mg and chicken would be 0.5 mg.

To treat PMS a daily dose of 50 mg of pyridoxine may be given, often with other B vitamins, from day ten of the menstrual cycle to day three of the following cycle. Alternatively, doses of between 100 to 200 mg may be taken throughout the menstrual cycle. At doses of over 500 mg taken for a long period, there may be damage to the nervous system resulting in clumsiness and unsteadiness, but these have not been found to occur in doses up to 200 mg. You don't need a prescription to buy pyridoxine over the counter, and it can be found at pharmacies or health food stores.

Vitamin E

Vitamin E is vital for healthy cell structure. It prolongs the life of red blood cells and slows down the ageing process. A deficiency would lead to the destruction of red blood cells which would result eventually in anaemia. Natural sources that are rich in this vitamin are extra virgin olive oil, cold pressed vegetable oils, wheatgerm and wholemeal cereals, and dark green leafy vegetables such as cabbage and spring greens. The recommended daily minimum requirement is 8 mg.

One hundred grams of wheatgerm will give you ten days' supply! If you eat a lot of polyunsaturated fats, you may need extra vitamin E since these work against each other, which is why low fat spreads and margarine often have vitamin E deliberately added to them. A normal healthy diet will contain sufficient vitamin E, but it is destroyed in foodstuffs by deep freezing and commercial food processing, which means that if most of your food is frozen or pre-prepared you may not be getting enough.

Vitamin E seems to be effective for some women in the relief of some of their PMS symptoms. This seems to be particularly so if anxiety or depression is the main problem. Vitamin E supplements are usually measured in International Units (IUs) and 15 IUs equals 10 mg. Doses of between 150 to 600 mg a day can be used and harmful effects are rare. Since vitamin E is fat-soluble, which means that it is absorbed by and stored in your body's fat, it can accumulate. At very high doses it can be harmful, leading to stomach pains, skin rashes, raised cholesterol levels and blood clots. You are more likely to have side effects if you take more than 250 mg a day for some time. It is available over the counter at your local pharmacy and health food store.

Magnesium

Magnesium is essential for healthy bones and teeth, and is important in helping your body turn blood sugar into energy. Magnesium helps your body to regulate its temperature, and is involved in passing along nerve impulses and the way your muscles contract. A deficiency in this mineral may lead to tremors in your hands, and even cramping spasms in the hands and feet. Magnesium deficiency can also be associated with anxiety and depression, irritability and memory loss. Because these symptoms are often found to be associated with PMS it has been theorised that a deficiency of magnesium might be involved, but studies have been inconclusive. It is also suggested that oestrogen therapy, including the Pill, can reduce the level of magnesium in the blood. Since some women say their PMS only developed when they went on the Pill or has got worse since being on it, the connection between magnesium and PMS has been made.

As with so many suggested treatments for PMS, magnesium supplements have certainly helped some people and are so worth trying. The recommended daily allowance for magnesium is 300 to 400 mg. It is mostly found in green leafy vegetables, nuts, wholemeal cereals, soya beans and seafoods. If you live in a hard water area you are also likely to get magnesium from your drinking water. Magnesium is available over the counter as a part of various multi-vitamin and mineral preparations. As long as there is nothing wrong with your kidneys there is very little risk involved in taking too much magnesium, although a very high increase could lead to nausea, vomiting and muscle weakness.

Zinc

Zinc plays a vital role in the activities of over a hundred enzymes in your body. Enzymes are the proteins that control chemical reactions in the body. For instance, the liver contains enzymes that break down nutrients and drugs, and your digestive tract contains enzymes that help digest food. Zinc is esssential for the production of the genetic material in your cells and helps your body use the carbohydrates you digest. A zinc deficiency may lead to a loss of appetite and a reduced sense of taste. A severe lack of zinc over a long period can lead to skin rashes and hair loss. Again, since these are symptoms of PMS, some clinicians have suggested there may be a link between PMS and zinc deficiency, and that therefore zinc preparations might help with PMS. Some sufferers do say they note an improvement so it's worth trying.

Recommended daily amounts are 15 mg and you usually find this in your daily diet. Zinc is found mostly in protein-rich food such as lean meat and seafood – a romantic meal of 100 mg of oysters would give you three days' supply! It is also found in wholemeal bread and cereals, and dried pulses. Zinc supplements are available over the counter either as a single ingredient or in multi-vitamin and mineral preparations. Long-term use of large doses of zinc can interfere with your body's absorption of iron and copper, two other essential minerals, and this could lead to headaches, nausea and vomiting. So you shouldn't take more than 15 mg a day without seeing a doctor.

Multi-vitamin preparations

As has already been suggested, increasing your intake of a particular vitamin or mineral can have an effect on the way your body deals with other elements. This is why it is often suggested that if you are taking a supplement it should be done as a combined preparation containing different vitamins and minerals, each balancing each other. Multi-vitamins are available over the counter at pharmacies or health food stores.

GLA (evening primrose oil)

Evening primrose oil contains a substance called gamma-linolenic acid (GLA). GLA encourages the body's ability to synthesise some prostaglandins. Prostaglandins are chemicals made by body tissue and have various roles. One of these is to sensitise pain receptors. When something goes wrong in your body and you need to be alerted to the fact that there is inflammation or some other problem, your body produces prostaglandins which cause you to feel pain or discomfort. Evening primrose oil has been suggested as particularly helping with PMS when symptoms include breast pain and bowel upsets. One suggestion is that it may be an upset in the balance between prostaglandins that causes premenstrual changes, rather than an increase in them. Taking evening primrose oil may allow your body to restore a balance. A suggested dose is between two to six 500 mg capsules twice a day after food, although some enthusiasts recommend up to eight. It is available over the counter as a single supplement or as part of a multi-vitamin and mineral preparation. Other natural sources of GLA are safflower oil, borage seed oil and black-currant seed oil.

PSYCHOTHERAPY

The psychotherapy approach involves counselling, advice and sympathy. The main aim is to remove any guilt or blame you may feel about the symptoms of your PMS or the behaviour they produce in you. The psychotherapy approach helps you to understand and accept that your behaviour or symptoms have a biochemical cause and are not due to your 'losing your mind' or having a defective personality. As many women who have tried this approach will testify gratefully, just being listened to and believed is often enough for a woman to be able to break the vicious circle of symptoms producing stress and stress causing further symptoms.

Part of any stress surrounding a woman who has PMS is the reaction, particularly if they are unsympathetic or critical, of others around her. The reactions of a partner can be the most important and influential of these, and seeking couple counselling can be extremely useful and rewarding. An informed and sympathetic partner can give the additional bonus of offering help and support in any drug, diet or exercise regimen that you are using, as well as hopefully taking on more of the domestic load of chores and responsibilities at the time when any of your PMS symptoms are most troublesome.

The most important part of counselling is for you to have a chance to listen to and understand yourself. It will probably be the first time that everything to do with your PMS has been gathered together in one place and examined by you. This will be the first chance you will have to get the

complete picture, rather than just sifting through discon-
nected fragments. You may be scornful about the idea that
what has happened in your past might be having a very
strong influence on your feelings and behaviour in the present. We tend to laugh at the idea that childhood experiences and our relationship with our parents might be at
the root of any discomfort we have now. But the fact is
that it can. Thinking and talking about the past, and its
relevance to the present, is certainly something you can
do on your own or with friends and family. However it's
difficult to be objective which is why making this journey
with a professional counsellor would probably be more
helpful to you. It has to be stressed that going the counselling route does not imply that PMS is imaginary or purely
emotional. Strong feelings do end up expressed in physical
terms. Deal with and come to terms with your emotions,
and you may well find your biochemistry alters
accordingly.

THE PLACEBO EFFECT

The effectiveness of coming to terms with your feelings or
gaining a feeling of being in control may be seen in the
effectiveness of the so-called placebo effect in PMS treatment. Many of the treatments suggested – progesterone,
evening primrose oil, diet etc. – have strong support from
women who swear by them. There is plenty of anecdotal
evidence to say that each of these treatments offers *the*
cure. However, these promises never seem to hold up in
scientific trials.

In a proper trial subjects would be matched and then
randomly given the treatment or the placebo. This is called
a 'double blind trial'. The doctor actually giving you the
treatment usually doesn't even know whether you are on
the active or placebo pills. Sometimes half way through

the trial the treatment will be switched so that women on the treatment will be given the placebo, and the other way round. This is called a 'double blind crossover trial'. Fairly obviously the results will usually be very different, depending on whether or when you were on the real thing or the sugar pill.

The problem with PMS trials is that the placebo is often found to be just as effective as the treatment being investigated – or just as ineffective. But what you could argue is that this shows how effective is the conviction that something helpful is being done. If you convince yourself that there is an answer that you've searched for and found, and that works, this doesn't mean that you are stupid or that your discomfort was imaginary. What it does show is that your feelings of being ignored or devalued were strong enough to make you physically ill, and that taking steps to do something about it and being listened to was important enough to you to make you feel better. In one controlled study, women who received help with making changes to their lives as well as drug treatment did far better than those just given tablets. Improvements in mood were maintained three months after the therapy – an oral progesterone – was stopped.

'I went to my doctor and he was really good. I was upset, and I was worried about taking up his time and he came out to the reception with me and asked them to make a special, long appointment for me the next afternoon. So I went in and he let me talk for ages. He gave me some pills, and said for me to do some exercise and gave me a relaxation tape. It got better but I still had problems and he tried some other pills, but they gave me a funny skin reaction. So he gave me a third lot of pills and they really did the trick. I felt miles better and I haven't had real problems for ages. I saw him recently, when I needed jabs for a foreign holiday and

I asked him what the pills he'd given me were, because my friend has PMS and she needs help. He said I should tell her to come and see him and he'd do the best he could. He said I shouldn't tell her, but the pills he gave me the last time didn't have anything in them. He reckoned it was me, and him listening to me, that really did the trick.'

Seeing a doctor for help with PMS may be your best route. But there is also a lot you can do for yourself, and there are treatments you may want to try that are not always available from a conventional medical practitioner. We will be looking at these in Chapter 10.

10

What else can be done?

LOOKING AFTER YOURSELF

One of the biggest barriers to dealing successfully with PMS, or any other condition for that matter, is frequently how we see ourselves, and how we seek treatment and deal with it once it has been offered. Women are far from being the weaker sex and have a longer life expectancy, and greater stamina and resistance to disease than men. But we also tend to neglect ourselves and be neglected by those around us. In general, the traditional female role of looking after everyone else before yourself means you come under greater strain than the men in your family, social and working life. Some indication of this is that when you compare the health of married women to married men, unmarried women and unmarried men, the worst off are the married women, while the best off are the married men.

In the last 25 years the number of women going out to work in the UK has increased to the point where women are some 50 per cent of the labour force, but there is little to show that men are increasing their share of domestic or child care duties to ease the additional workload. Instead, the majority of women carry a double or even triple burden, working both in and outside the home, and their health, their well-being and the amount of time they can 'afford' to deal with their own ills often suffers as a result.

> 'I just haven't got the time to go to my doctor. I can't make an appointment in the day because getting time off work isn't practical. There's a limit to the number of times you can have off for hospital or doctors' appointments, and I have to go easy on asking for them because I know the children will need to go some time or other. I can't go in the evening because surgery is always full, and if you take the children with you they get bored and kick up a fuss, and you can't leave them at home without a sitter, and sitters cost money. My husband works late so he can't look after them, and even if he was there, I'd get home to fights and a mess so I'd rather just leave it.'

Women tend to neglect their health and it can be hard to appreciate how much influence we can have over our own well-being. What most of us need to do to improve our lives enormously is to *make* the time we need to look after ourselves, too. It only takes the understanding that you can have a surprisingly significant effect on yourself to give you the motivation to do this, and a bit of information to give you the confidence to start. There are, however, many barriers to good health care for women. The most obvious one is the lack of time. There is often little of this left after home, children, partner and work have taken their share, and we are still brought up to think that a woman who takes time out to care for herself is being selfish and taking this time away from those she should be looking after.

The reality is that there is time to spare. What causes the false shortage is the inherited belief that any free time should be spent on truly important things, and that women and their health do not fall into this category. Women are not the only ones who feel this. Often the very people, the doctors, who should be helping them, share this view. A commonly reported complaint by women is that some male doctors still make us feel that our visits to the surgery are time-wasting, or that our complaints are neurotic, trivial or, worst of all, simply 'female'.

The intention of this chapter is to explain as many as possible of the further treatments that are available for PMS. Equally important to trying a specific treatment or therapy is to recognise and accept that for any particular part of your body to remain healthy, or for a specific condition to be cured or alleviated, the whole body must be functioning as well as it can. This is known as the 'holistic' approach and for it to work you need to consider everything in your lifestyle. This includes not just your medical health, but also diet, leisure, work, relationships and the environment in which these all take place. The more we know about ourselves and how the various elements in our life can affect us, the better opportunities we will have to make these effects good ones. You can do a lot for yourself, without necessarily needing a doctor's help.

BEING SUPERWOMAN

Most women suffer from a common delusion. We are trained from birth to think that everything is down to us. We have to look after everyone else – our friends, our parents, our partners, our family. Women are brought up to feel there is something horribly selfish and horribly sinful in ever caring for our own needs. Everyone else must come first and that means that we rarely even get a chance to put ourselves second. We simply don't figure in the equation at all. It is easy to see then why PMS may actually have more to do with an emotional or stress-related reaction than a purely physical cause. Saying it is PMS that makes us angry, weepy or downright uncooperative gives you a chance to say 'No'. You can have your own way but without being unfeminine enough to own up to the fact that you don't want to do what everyone is demanding or expecting you to do.

Without in any way suggesting that the symptoms and discomfort you experience are 'all in the mind', I am suggesting that you might find an improvement in your wellbeing if you were able to face up to and own any negative feelings or anger that you have. You don't have to be the perfect daughter, friend, partner or parent. There are times when it is perfectly acceptable for the house to be a mess, for the family to get their own supper, and for you to lock the bathroom door and to have an hour's soak in the tub with a book and without a guilty conscience.

In Chapter 9 we saw how it might be helpful to talk to a sympathetic and experienced professional to help you get your feelings about yourself and your life in perspective. You can also do this for yourself and on your own. It is useful when you are feeling out of control and put upon, to sit down and work out your priorities. You can't do everything and it is totally unreasonable to think that you should. What is reasonable is to consider what is your responsibility, to hand back to others what they should be doing and to cut down on the amount of work that can reasonably be laid at your door.

'I must have spent loads of money trying to treat my PMS. I bought all the cures possible and none of them seemed to do much good. What made all the difference in the world was a friend of mine who told me I was an idiot to let my family get away with so much. All I did was put my foot down and got them all to pull their weight around the house. I said they had to do chores. They had to keep their own rooms tidy and if clothes weren't put in the basket or the washing machine they wouldn't be washed. Well, of course, the first month or so I gave in and it went on being the way it always was. But then I hardened up. One night, there were no coffee mugs downstairs and I had mine, but no one else did. They were all in the children's rooms, or out in the garage. When my partner started in, I said it wasn't down to me. So they all had to scout round the house and find them all, and wash them up! I felt so good, telling them it wasn't my job to run after them all the time. They pull their weight now or else, and I can honestly say I don't have PMS the way I used to.'

SELF-HELP

Suggesting that self-help could help in the treatment of PMS should not be misunderstood. I do not mean that PMS is some minor ailment, that only needs a bit of 'pulling yourself together' to have it disappear. What it should suggest is that there are many elements in every woman's life where some extra care, action or adjustment of behaviour could make real and sometimes lasting differences to the way in which PMS impacts on your life.

It is easy to assume that our health or lack of it, and whether we have such conditions as PMS, is something that simply happens to us. We treat such things as if they are nothing to do with our behaviour or lifestyle. These sorts of beliefs are understandable, but they are also very unhelpful to us. There is a lot of evidence to suggest a relationship between ill-health and the way we live. This is not to say that you can banish ill-health by 'pulling up your socks' or that being ill is in any way your fault. But it does suggest that taking control and being self-determining may help you.

EXTRA HELP

Assertiveness training

One of the best ways of helping yourself work out what is and what is not your responsibility is a course of assertiveness training. Being assertive is not the same as being aggressive. If you are assertive you don't always get your own way. What you do learn is the ability to be clear about what you can and can't do, and how to put that across to other people in a way that leaves everyone feeling good about it. You can find our from your local library or adult education centre about assertiveness groups in your area. An assertiveness course usually consists of six to ten sessions with a group of like-minded people led by an experienced trainer.

Self-help groups

We all need support. You might already have a sympathetic group of friends or family and find it easy to get together with them for a good moan and a session of boosting each other's self-esteem. If this doesn't happen in your life, then there are ways of finding just such a set of people. There are self-help groups for all sorts of specific situations, or women's groups that are simply there to put women in touch with each other for mutual encouragement. Again, ask at your local library or adult education centre to see what is available near you.

IMPROVING THINGS

So, what are these factors that make for well-being or lack of it, and how can you best help yourself by influencing them? Important areas to look at are your eating, drinking and smoking habits, your general fitness, your ability to deal with stress and the environment in which you live, work and play. Any or all of these can be instrumental in deciding whether you do or do not meet difficulties, and all of them are factors which you can change or affect to improve your life.

Eating

Food cravings

PMS and food seem to have a specific relationship. Food cravings are frequently a particular symptom. A high proportion of women who report having premenstrual discomfort will say that it shows itself in an irresistible longing for salty or sweet foods, particularly chocolate. Others will say that they find themselves drawn to pasta or other starchy snacks in the premenstruum. Several studies have suggested that not only do women with PMS eat more calories premenstrually, but their preference for certain foods and even their taste sensitivity changes at this time.

Premenstrual food cravings often go hand-in-hand with mood changes. One suggestion is that they share a cause – an alteration in brain chemistry. Depression, particularly when it is serious depressive illness, is usually associated with a loss of appetite. But there is another disorder in which sadness and 'the munchies' go together. This is seasonal affective disorder or SAD. SAD has been shown to happen when sufferers react to the lack of light experienced in the long nights and short days of winter by a chemical imbalance that produces depression. One argument is that the same sort of imbalance happens to PMS sufferers and that it can be reversed by altering the diet. Eating carbohydrates will trigger a release of insulin into your body and this allows an amino acid called tryptophan to act on your brain, increasing the production and release of another chemical called 5-HT. If you don't have enough of this chemical available in your brain, this can lead to depression.

Carbohydrate increases this effect but protein decreases it, so it is starchy food that helps. That means eating more potatoes, rice, corn, bread or any other grain product such as crackers or pitta.

Just as pain is the way your body tells you it has sustained some damage and you had better do something about it, food cravings may have a similar good explanation. A pregnant woman's longing to nibble lumps of coal or a PMS sufferer's desire for chocolate may actually be a pretty reasonable attempt to draw attention to the fact that something essential is lacking and needed. The difficulty, of course, is that we sometimes get these messages confused.

Food is nearly always associated in our minds with comfort. This is hardly surprising since our earliest memories will have been of the bliss we experienced as babies when the pains of hunger and loneliness were banished in the arms of a comforting, loving and food-giving parent. Food equals love, so at times when we need a bit of love and comfort we turn to it. We also often associate sweet food particularly with care and attention – a link usually forged in our minds by the presents, rewards or bribes given to us as children. The danger here, then, is that when we experience a food craving which is actually for a substance that may help our physical symptoms, we may eat something that could give us a psychological boost but has no effect on the body itself or actually has the wrong one. However, this is where the complex mind/body interface can cause problems. While some studies show that carbohydrate can be used to deal effectively with both food cravings and depression in PMS sufferers, other studies show that satisfying the longing, far from lifting your mood, can make you feel even more depressed afterwards. The suggestion here is that some women would feel satisfied, strong and in control if they resisted their food cravings, and having given in to them, soon after are depressed at their failure.

The other problem with satisfying cravings with a quick intake of sugar is that the initial surge of satisfaction is quickly countered by an equal drop. This can lead very quickly to a cycle where you keep eating chocolate or other sweets because you feel depressed or hungy – a depression or hunger that has actually been caused by your earlier intake! The medical explanation for this cycle is that the sugar goes rapidly into your bloodstream and gives an immediate increase in your blood sugar level. Your body releases insulin to cope with this, which forces the blood sugar level down and also produces a surge of adrenaline. This is the hormone that gets you on your toes and wakes you up . . . and increases your appetite!

The PMS diet

Three-hourly snacks

One suggested treatment for PMS is a strict regime of three-hourly starch snacks. This means that you have to have some carbohydrate, if only a slice of toast or a cracker, every three hours, making sure you eat something within an hour of going to sleep and immediately you wake up. If you try this regime, you do need to be very organised, carry supplies with you and keeping an eye on the time. You need to have the self-confidence to be able to interrupt whatever you are doing and to pull out your carbohydrate snack if your three hours are up! Enthusiasts of this treatment say it is effective, but only if you follow it to the letter. Being at all late in eating will throw you back into suffering symptoms, they say. Keep to it, and it will work, they promise.

The interesting point about a diet like this is that it actually puts you into the eating regime that our grand-parents would have taken for granted. That is, breakfast followed by 'elevenses' and a lunch at one o'clock. Tea between three and four would have set you up for an evening meal at some time around six or seven with a light supper just before bedtime. If you accept the idea that PMS is a modern condition, you can't help won-dering whether our present-day way of eating might have something to do with it. War-time rationing, fol-lowed by worries about diet, led the last two generations to become committed to the idea of three square meals a day with snacking in between as somehow unhealthy. The result often is that we *do* snack, because our bodies kick up a fuss otherwise, but we snack in a sneaky, disorganised way on foods with a high sugar content, such as chocolate bars, soft drinks and biscuits, with their attendant problems.

More recent advice for a healthy diet is that we should return to the way our ancestors probably ate and the way that our bodies are designed to best deal with food. This is effectively by 'grazing', or eating small and satis-fying amounts of food throughout the day, rather than saving them up for three binges. The idea is to eat the same amount as you may have been used to having as breakfast, lunch and an evening meal, but to do it either as six, or even more, mini meals. You may end up consuming fewer rather than more calories, because you don't eat extra calories in the shape of between-meal snacks. Done properly you would be eating a healthy and well-balanced diet which eliminates food cravings. You could see it as a treatment for PMS, but equally you could see it as a natural system of eating for any member of the family.

Fresh is best

If you want to change your eating pattern, the first and main principle of healthy eating is that fresh is best. What you should be trying to do is reduce the amount of salt, fat and sugar you eat. One dramatic way of doing so is to get rid of the hidden extra amounts found in refined and pre-prepared dishes. Avoid saturated fats – that means butter, margarine, fat spreads (even the ones that say they are low-fat) and lard. Instead, use cold-pressed vegetable oils such as extra virgin olive oil. Cut down, or even cut out, red meat, and if you do eat it make sure you trim off all visible fat. Don't forget that cheaper meat products such as sausages or pies are usually less expensive because they use a large proportion of the cheaper fat to lean meat. If you don't want to go the whole 'hog' and become a veget-arian, at least increase the proportion of white meat, such as chicken and fish, to red meat you eat. Interestingly, a lot of people who start off reducing the amount of red meat they eat as a part of weight control or because of problems such as PMS do find their tastes change. Go for the 'five a day' fruit and vegetable rule, and eat at least five portions of fruit, vegetables and/or salad every day, with a particu-lar emphasis on leafy green vegetables such as cabbage or sprouts.

There have been studies suggesting that PMS may be associated with, or worsened by, caffeine, although the results are not conclusive. However, the fact is that, just as with saturated fats, sugar and salt, there is plenty of evid-ence to say all these substances are bad for your health. Whether they cause or worsen PMS symptoms or not, they do increase your risks of plenty of other health problems such as heart disease. For all these reasons, anyone who suffers from PMS could try cutting down on the amount of tea or coffee they take, or change to herbal teas and decaffeinated coffee.

If PMS is related to vitamin or mineral deficiencies, a healthy pattern of eating is the best way of dealing with this. Everyone, not only women and not only PMS sufferers, should reduce the amount of sugar, alcohol, caffeine and salt in their diet, eat balanced meals, eliminate nicotine and other recreational drugs, and exercise. You will be bound to notice an improvement in your general health as well as in PMS symptoms, not because dietary deficiencies cause the PMS or changes cure it, but because feeling good about yourself and in control is in itself beneficial, both physically and emotionally.

Being overweight

We have just considered the special and specific dietary considerations and requirements for a PMS sufferer. What we still need to look at is the more general picture of our daily eating patterns. What and how you eat can be one of the most important factors in whether or not you are basically healthy, or are likely to have problems or worsen any you already have. Simply being overweight can put strain on your heart and increase your blood pressure. It can then bring further problems by putting extra stresses on your joints that can bring on arthritis in later years. Being overweight can also act on the hormone system and could therefore add particular complications for a woman with PMS.

The difficulty with dealing with being overweight is that the whole matter of a woman's shape and body size is clouded by social attitudes and pressures to conform to some sort of ideal. More and more women are quite rightly reacting against these pressures to be slim for purely cosmetic reasons, but if you do choose to be considerably overweight, you should at least recognise that you are also choosing to risk a wide range of health problems.

If you see yourself as being overweight and would like

to change, perhaps the first step is to accept that aiming for a realistic weight that will give you health benefits is far better than going for some idealised goal you will never reach. All this second approach is likely to do is give you a sense of failure and so stop you persisting with the healthier eating changes you had introduced into your life. Whatever you see as your target, trying to get there through one more magic, easy diet is unlikely to help you very much. This is because diets often do not focus on the central issue, which is that far too many of us eat too much fat, too much sugar, and not enough fresh foods and fibre. Too many of us then compound our bad habits by not exercising as much as we should.

If you become a 'dieter', you are likely to see-saw between strict, low-calorie regimens, alternating with treats in the form of cakes and chips and the like. To get it right, and to get the satisfying and health-giving result you want, see the word 'diet' as meaning your everyday pattern of eating, instead of a hard, self-denying and short-term purgatory. Changing your eating patterns does not mean giving up the pleasures of eating. You can stop using large quantities of dangerous and unhealthy stuff, and still enjoy daily menus that are as varied as your old eating habits.

It could be argued that the so-called PMS diet is not more than a healthy way of eating that would make anybody – male or female, PMS sufferer or non-sufferer – feel better. It may work, not only because it helps you feel on top of and in control of yourself and your life, but because it is the natural, best and healthiest way of managing your nutrition.

Drinking

Changing our drinking habits to benefit our health is, for most people, even harder than trying to do something about how and what they eat. Drink is almost an automatic part of most of our social life and there seem to be more do than don't attitudes about its use. Our doctors largely agree that moderate wine consumption may be good for the heart and the circulation. Even the Bible can be used in support of this view when it says 'Take a little wine for thy stomach's sake and thine often infirmities.' In this atmosphere, it can be very easy to go over the sensible limits – the point beyond which 'moderate' slips into the unhealthy, and on towards the downright damaging and dangerous. What can surprise most people, who have previously not questioned the amount or the frequency with which they drink, is how low the level is at which the experts think you start to do damage to your body and your life.

The safe drinking limit for women is no more than 13 units of drink a week. A unit is half a pint of beer, a single pub optic measure of spirits (note here that any spirit drinks you have at home tend to be in much bigger measures than this), or a standard-sized glass of wine, sherry or fortified wine. If you have a partner, it might be easier to change your drinking habits if he looks at his drinking at the same time as you look at yours. The average man can drink a little more than the average women because of his greater size and a slightly different body composition. The general rule is that men can drink two or three *pints* or their equivalent two or three times a week, and that women can have two or three *units* two or three times a week to keep within a fairly safe limit.

Any more than these limits and the first thing that suffers is your waistline. After that, there are increasingly damaging results, even though the drinking has not become 'heavy' or a problem in itself. What sort of harm can it cause? Some medical research suggests that as little as three glasses of wine a week increases a woman's risks of developing breast cancer by 50 per cent (Rosenburg et al., 1982). There are also studies which suggest that alcohol may have a link with PMS (Kato et al., 1989). You may take a drink or two to help you over the stresses of PMS, but the chances are that some of your sumptoms are worsened or even encouraged by alcohol consumption.

Smoking

No one can argue against the fact that smoking is bad for your health. As well as increasing your chances of developing lung cancer, it can also increase your risk of developing cancer of the cervix. However, smoking not only has general health risks, but also a negative pay-off for anyone reading this book since it is suggested that women smokers are more likely to suffer from PMS.

If you are a woman smoker, you will also go into menopause around two years earlier than a non-smoker, but this is not an advantage. Menopause may put paid to PMS, but it brings on all sorts of health risks such as osteoporosis and heart disease. And, while you are puffing your way towards all these misfortunes, you will not look so good either. Smokers suffer from more facial wrinkles than non-smokers, so much so that this condition is referred to as 'smoker's face', and many doctors claim they can tell if a patient is a smoker simply by looking at them. If you smoke on, in spite of all the evidence against the habit, after menopause you will be far more likely to suffer from osteoporosis as your bones lose their calcium, and become brittle and easily broken.

Remember also that any level of cigarette smoking increases not only your own health risks but those of your children as well. It has been established, for example, that children of smokers have a higher risk of suffering bronchial and other illnesses. The dangers of 'passive smoking' – inhaling someone else's cigarette smoke – are beginning to be understood and confirmed, and more and more workplaces and public areas are helping the majority who do not smoke to avoid this dangerous nuisance. So, just as you should not smoke yourself, you should also have the confidence to assert your right to clean lungs and do your bit to have the habit banned in as many places as possible, be it in your own house, at work or in public places.

If actually giving up is your problem, then your doctor would be only too delighted to help you. In addition, there is a wide range of free leaflets and inexpensive books to give you support, as well as some excellent self-help groups. If you would like to make your workplace a no-smoking area, and your employer has not already taken this initiative, contact your union representative or the local health and safety officer for advice.

Exercise

Exercise may not only be a factor in good health. It may also have some particular benefits in coping with the treating of PMS in that it improves muscle tone, and so relieves aches and reduces tension. Regular exercise can be enormously beneficial for anyone suffering PMS, helping you feel physically better, as well as improving self-esteem and self-confidence. It doesn't matter what sort of exercise you do as long as it is vigorous and gets you puffed – energetic walking, running, cycling, keep fit, step or other conditioning classes, or even weight training. What is important is that you do it regularly. Two or three sessions a week may make a marked improvement.

'I hated the idea of exercise. I was awful at sports at school. My friend goes to a gym in town and she was always on at me to go along too, but I wouldn't. I knew I should be doing more exercise but I just didn't want to go. They had an open night so I went along to shut her up, and because they had a free glass of wine on offer and it was an hour or two out with friends. I couldn't have been more surprised. They did a demonstration class and everyone was so friendly, especially the woman who runs the place. I've been going to step classes for a year now, twice a week. I've lost a stone, I feel terrific and it's a real break. You can go in feeling tired and fed up and you come out feeling on top of the world.'

Environment

It will invalidate a lot of any efforts we may make to look after ourselves generally, and tackle PMS specifically, if we don't consider our living and working conditions as part of the general formula. It's no use giving up the dreadful weed, drinking sensibly, eating correctly and getting lots of healthy exercise if we do all or some of these things in conditions which in themselves can be positively damaging to our well being..

Whether you work in or outside the home you should check to see if you are being affected by any of the physical, biological, psychological or chemical influences which could harm you in some way. Some of the physical hazards to look for would be excess noise, poor lighting, radiation, excessive temperatures, repetitive movements that can cause muscular strain, and working conditions or your own working methods that demand the lifting of too heavy weights or of remaining standing for extended periods. The chemical hazards, both at work and home, can come from dust, fumes, gases and vapours, chemical liquids and solids, and we can be subjected to biological hazards from germs, dirty conditions or from contact with infected materials. Finally, in any check of whether or not your living and working conditions are acceptable, don't forget to consider if there are any psychological hazards coming from stress, boredom, overwork or harassment that could be removed or reduced in your lifestyle.

TAKING ACTION

In the best of all possible worlds for a woman, she would be able to be an easy-going non-smoker who only has the odd glass or so with her carefully chosen low-fat diet, which she eats between her regular visits to her gym for her exercise sessions. She would also have a home or a working life where she was completely free from contact with anything that could be hazardous to her health in any way. However, if the Good Lord in all her wisdom has not placed you in this particular ideal state, what can you realistically do for yourself and how can you arrange your life around good health?

First, you could start to accept the idea that you are what you eat, and that how we view and treat food probably cause more problems to women than anything else. This will probably apply just as much whether you live on your own or are a mother looking after the feeding of a husband and family. Either way, most women have some sorts of pressures that dictate and affect the way they buy, cook and serve food in their daily lives. It might be money, it might be time or it might be the fads and foibles of the people we eat with. This last point can be a particularly strong influence if any attempt to cook and serve 'healthy' food is met only with whines, complaints and waste from a husband or family whose unshakeable argument is simply that they don't like it. Whatever the source of any pressures against change, the chances are that most women will have found that the easiest course is to go on turning out the fatty and sugary foods that the family will eat, over the more nutritious elements everyone really needs.

If you really want to increase your long-term chances of

becoming and staying healthy, and tackle your PMS, you really have to opt for, and maybe even have to fight for, a healthy diet. This will mean using fewer prepared and packaged foods, and making more use of fresh and high fibre foods such as wholemeal bread and pasta. It will also require taking a little more time and care in shopping and preparation, the main idea here being to seek out the bargains in seasonal fruit and vegetables, meat and fish, and to then make them into attractive meals to both satisfy yourself and gain the support of your family in your efforts towards healthy eating.

Often we have a preference for the unhealthy fatty, sweet food because we've never really examined our eating patterns. In fact, for many people it is no more than a habit, rather than because the healthier alternative is actually less tasty or attractive. Fresh flavours can seem a bit bland at first after the less subtle tastes of artificial flavours, but if you can hold out against the initial howls and complaints of your own taste buds and those of your family, you will probably find that healthier food soon becomes preferable, as well. A bonus in your efforts to eat well is that you don't have to fight the good fight on your own. Most doctors are now only too happy to help, knowing the risks of being overweight and eating badly can only result in more unwanted complications and work for them.

Putting healthier calories into your body will not be enough in itself. Adequate exercise is also called for to make up the healthy whole. Just as there are strategies for successfully introducing good eating patterns into your life, so there are keys to letting exercise do something for you. The chief among these is to start slowly, monitor your progress continually and gradually increase your efforts until you reach the level which is best for you to gain and maintain your fitness. It will help to work out whether you need company and encouragement to get anything done, or if you would be happier doing things on your own. If you feel that your good intentions may waver without the moral support of others, then join a class or group in your local leisure centre, at an evening class or gym. If there is no keep fit class near you, start your own! Getting together with a group of like-minded friends and neighbours to exercise to music or go jogging will do wonders for your general well-being, and quite a bit for your social life as well.

RELAXATION

If you accept that either PMS is a stress-related condition or that at least PMS symptoms are made worse by the stress you feel at having them, you will see that some form of relaxation is likely to help. There are many ways of relieving tension. Yoga, PFT, relaxation exercises, massage and aromatherapy are some of them.

Yoga

Yoga is an ancient Indian tradition combining breathing exercises, stretching and concentration to promote relaxation and calmness of mind. You can learn from a book or video how to do it yourself, but it is probably best done in a class led by an experienced teacher. Although you may have the impression that you need rubber joints to do yoga, it is actually suitable for anyone, no matter how inflexible or unfit you may be to start with.

PFT

PFT is a wonderful American term. It's short for pet facilit-ated therapy! Serious research has shown that keeping animals can have a quite dramatic effect on the well-being, both emotional and physical, of their owners. Stroking a furry animal, talking to a pet or watching the graceful movements of fish can actually lower blood pressure and relieve stress. Those few days before your period arrives may be a particularly good time to take the dog for a walk or curl up with a cat and a hot water bottle, and indulge in a bout of PFT. Your pet will like it and so will you.

De-stressing exercises

Relaxation isn't just a case of sitting down with a cup of coffee – the coffee, unless it's decaffeinated, will spoil the effect anyway! Often, when we take a break, we spend it worrying or planning what we are going to do next, so the time is hardly spent unwinding. What you need, to really relax, is to let go of anything that is bothering you and to allow your body muscles to lose their tension. One way of doing this is to count down slowly, from ten to one, moving through your body from your head to your feet, first tensing and then fully letting go each and every muscle in your body on the way. You can get relaxation tapes that will talk you through this process, which is a form of self-hypnosis, and which will help you de-stress in as little as ten minutes.

Massage

Shiatsu massage involves pressing or stroking the points very similar to those stimulated in acupuncture and it has much the same effect. But simply pressing and stroking skin and muscles can make you feel good. Massage may have this effect by loosening tight and tense muscles, and encouraging blood flow, or it simply may be that it feels comforting and soothing to be touched. You can learn how to massage from books and videos. To start, make sure you are warm and won't be disturbed. Spread a towel or sheet on somewhere comfortable yet firm – a bed, sofa or even the floor –

and lie down. Your partner takes a handful of oil or cream and proceeds to smooth it over you. As this is done, you will discover what makes you feel good. Direct them to areas that need relaxing – your back, neck and shoulders, perhaps, or forehead and temples. You may find having your feet and hands manipulated is surprisingly pleasant. Some women find massage around the small of the back and the belly is particularly helpful at this time in the month but others say it is painful and puts them on edge. You can massage yourself, as well, but it is far more effective and relaxing if you can get someone else to do it for you.

Aromatherapy

Aromatherapy is massage with an extra. When you have an ordinary massage, the masseur will use oil or cream on their hands to help them glide over your body easily and comfortably. In aromatherapy, concentrated essential oils are added to the basic carrier oil. Oils, ranging from lavender, camomile and rosemary to basil, will each, separately and in combination, be used to different effect. Jasmine, ylang-ylang and geranium are all said to be excellent for depression. Orange blossom, patchouli and sandalwood can help with tension, and clary sage, marjoram and rose will have a sedative effect.

Aromatherapy probably has a complex action. Not only is the massage obviously soothing, but the oils themselves work in different ways. Scents have quite a dramatic effect on mood. But more than that, although skin is largely designed to be waterproof, and you shouldn't believe everything cosmetic ads tell you about substances being absorbed, there is no doubt chemicals put on the skin can seep through into the bloodstream.

We now give drugs by skin patches, and the fact is that when you swallow a drug it has to go through the stomach and liver which can reduce any effect considerably. A small amount can go a long way when it's absorbed directly into the bloodstream.

ACUPUNCTURE

The ancient Chinese art of acupuncture is said to be over 5,000 years old. Needles are stuck into the skin at specific points. The Chinese describe around a thousand of these points. The needle or needles, which are very light and thin, are inserted and left for anything between a few seconds to several minutes. The acupuncturist usually rotates or vibrates the needles between their fingertips and some practitioners even do this with a very small electric current. It sounds painful, but in fact it is not because the needles only penetrate a few millimetres and are so very thin the patient very rarely feels anything other than the relief this treatment can provide.

For a long time Western science believed that acupuncture worked as a sort of faith healing where the patient improved because they believed in the treatment. However, since acupuncture has been shown to work on unconscious patients and on animals it came to be accepted that there was likely to be a real reaction. The Chinese explain that *chi*, or body energy, circulates through meridians or pathways in the body and that ill-health happens when an imbalance occurs. Acupuncture, they say, restores the proper flow. Western medicine suggests that acupuncture stimulates the release of endorphins and encephalins, which are natural painkillers in the body, similar to morphine. It is the same thing, only using a different language!

Acupuncture seems to be particularly helpful therefore in conditions involving anxiety, stress, tension and chronic pain, which is why it may well be useful for PMS. There is plenty of anecdotal evidence that it can be useful, but no controlled studies, and the effect would seem to vary from person to person. Some people may find it relieves symptoms after a short course of treatment and that this improvement is maintained. Others may find it certainly helps, but they need to have regular sessions, often just before PMS symptoms usually start. It is now available on the NHS in many health centres and hospital physiotherapy departments. Ask your doctor.

REFLEXOLOGY

Reflexology is another ancient Chinese therapy, akin to acupuncture. It involves deep massage of the soles of the feet and sometimes the hands. The idea is that areas of the foot share the same nerve supplies as organs in the rest of the body. So, for instance, an area under the arch of the foot relates to the stomach. The theory is that massaging this area will stimulate and affect the stomach, and that this area would be tender if you had any problems in the stomach. Treatment involves the patient lying comfortably while the reflexologist gently presses and strokes the feet, first diagnosing the problem and then applying the massage to treat it. As with acupuncture, it is likely that the stimulation of massage encourages the body's own defences to deal with particular conditions.

Reflexologists claim good results with many chronic conditions, particularly migraine and other headaches, and stress-related illnesses. For that reason reflexology may indeed be worth trying for PMS. There are no controlled studies on the subject, but anecdotal evidence that it has helped some people.

HOMOEOPATHY

Homoeopathy is only around 200 years old but is based on ideas that go back to Hippocrates, the Greek physician who lived 2,500 years ago and who is said to be the father of medicine. Homoeopathy is founded on the idea of 'like treating like'. Homoeopaths will take a substance that produces particular symptoms when taken in excess and use it to treat exactly that symptom. Homoeopaths also believe that when diluted by an extraordinary amount, a substance's power to cure is increased while its harmful side-effects disappear. Since by the time the full process is completed only a few molecules of the original substance are left in the remedy that is offered to you, science cannot really explain why homoeopathy may work, but it certainly does for many people.

One explanation could be that homoeopathy is best when offered by an experienced homoeopath who first takes a detailed history. Homoeopathy is supposed to be a 'whole person' medicine so it's important to take everything into account – details about your home and work life, your family and relationships, as well as the exact symptoms that are bothering you. The same symptom in two people may therefore be treated with different remedies. It could be argued that the opportunity for this concentrated, sympathetic face-to-face talk which usually takes an hour and a half, and is so very different from the six minutes allotted by the average GP, is what actually helps.

Homoeopathy remedies are available over the counter at pharmacists and health shops. You can find a registered homoeopathist through the British Homoeopathic Association, and more and more National Health general practitioners are offering it too.

HERBALISM

Herbalism is without doubt the first original branch of medicine. We can prove that plants were used to heal at least 60,000 years ago and undoubtedly herbal remedies have been known for longer than that. Herbalism, however, has quite a bad press, and is often considered to be cranky and unreliable. The reasons for this are probably that originally the tribal elders most knowledgeable and skilled in this art were women. When men decided to get into the act it became necessary for them to cast doubt on their rivals' skills and they've been doing that ever since. One argument for the efficacy of herbal medicines is that, being made from plants or extracts from plants, what you get is a compound therapy. This is much gentler than the sort of pure, single substance that is made in a laboratory.

As with homoeopathic remedies, there are herbal remedies that could be taken for various PMS symptoms. Dandelion leaf, for instance, is a powerful diuretic and in France is called *Pis-en-lit* or 'pee in the bed'. Fennel tea is also often suggested as a diuretic when you feel bloated. Camomile or limeflower tea have a calming effect, and are good for insomnia, and lemon balm lifts depression and stress. As with homoeopathy you can self-treat, but visiting a herbalist has the additional benefits of tailoring treatment percisely for you and giving you the chance for a heart-to-heart with someone who makes the time to listen to you. Herbal remedies are now available at many pharmacies, health food shops and from registered herbalists.

These are the treatments that are usually suggested as being helpful for PMS. There are many other therapies which you may find suit you. It may be worth experimenting with these and any others that sound appealing.

The obvious question that most people ask when faced with this bewildering array of possible therapies is which is the best. The answer has to be whichever suits you and which you would be happiest at not only trying, but sticking with. Working out which may be the best method for you is the subject of Chapter 11.

11

What suits you?

'WHICH TREATMENT IS BEST FOR ME?'

With such a bewildering number of possible treatments to try you could be forgiven for wondering 'Where do I start?' The question most people ask, of course, is which treatment is best? The problem here is that there is no simple answer. When it comes to PMS you will hear from a lot of different people who will swear by one treatment or regime and often belittle all the others. The fact is that no one treatment has a perfect record – or even a good record at treating the majority of people who try it. More than any other health difficulty, PMS appears to be so very individual that each person may well have to design their own treatment package. In other words, you are going to have to pick-and-mix until you find what works for you.

Before you even begin to consider treatment for PMS, first make sure that this *is* your problem. Using the advice in Chapter 6, keep a diary for at least three months. At the same time it would be worth while noting honestly what you eat and when, how much alcohol you drink, if you smoke how much, and detailing whether you exercise and how. Write down what's going on in your personal life and at work as well. Are you or have you been under any particular pressure, are there any events that might have put a particular stress on you or that might have reminded you of an important happening in the past? All this will help to work out if PMS is the problem and, whether it is or not, aid you in doing something about your difficulties.

At the same time as you are keeping your diary, you can try some of the self-help measures, including any of the nutritional supplements. After all, if they do work there is no point in your suffering any longer than necessary. Even if you feel able to go to your doctor at an early stage and give a clear description of your PMS, he or she is going to ask you to show a record of your symptoms over three to six months. So it may be helpful to have been keeping this diary for at least a month before you approach your GP. When you see your GP you and he or she together can consider the next stage.

SEEING YOUR DOCTOR

When you see a doctor you will need to be prepared for the sort of medical approach that you are likely to be offered. If you are really unlucky you may encounter a doctor who is unable to take PMS and your cry for help seriously – who won't listen, won't give you time and is likely to fob you off with suggestions to take painkillers, antidepressants or to pull yourself together. Such GPs are fortunately becoming rarer, but you do need to be aware that GPs frequently see women complaining of PMS and know from bitter experience that it is not an easy condition to treat. As soon as the ugly spectre of PMS raises its head their hearts are likely to sink. So, if your GP heaves a heavy sigh or their eyes glaze over, don't take it personally. It's just the awful prospect of being asked for much needed help that they may not be able to offer that gets him or her down. This means that it's important that the two of you cooperate and work as hard as possible in order to make your search for help successful.

If you feel that your GP isn't being helpful, don't put up with this sort of treatment. You have the right to ask to be taken on to another doctor's list and you don't have to give your reason for moving. Although, of course, it might help nudge an unsympathetic GP in cleaning up their act if you give your reason for taking your custom elsewhere. You can find a GP who is more helpful about PMS by asking around your friends to see if any of them have one who is sympathetic. You can also interview GPs by asking for an appointment to discuss their attitudes before considering signing on with them. You will also now find that nearly every GP or health practice produces a practice leaflet and this may well tell you if there is a PMS or women's clinic held by one of the doctors.

As I have already said in Chapter 6, it's really important for you to be clear and truthful when keeping a menstrual diary. Your GP will also go through your various symptoms, not only finding out when they occur but also what they are, how long they last and how severe they are. Your doctor is also likely to want to do a physical examination which will probably include an internal. This will be to check on your general health and also to find out if anything may be discovered that could point to a different reason for your symptoms, such as endometriosis, cysts or conditions such as diabetes or kidney problems. Your doctor is also likely to weigh you and to ask for some information on what you eat normally, whether you do any exercise, and whether you smoke or drink.

If you are going to your doctor believing that PMS is purely a physical condition you may find some of the other questions that could be asked impertinent or irrelevant. They are neither, because a doctor isn't prying or implying that you are being silly if he or she then goes on to discuss some details about your work life, your home life, your family and your relationships. Neither is it either dismissive or unreasonable for them to want to know if you've suffered from depression or any other emotional difficulty in the past.

Once your doctor and you have a clear picture of what has led up to your visit, the two of you can begin to consider doing something about it. But don't forget that quite a few of the treatments, such as danazol, oestrogen and psychotherapy, need some time to work. In a situation where you are not sure what causes the problem and what may help, you may have to try several solutions, giving each a fair trial, before finding one that works for you. You may need to accept that it could take up to a year before a solution is found.

It is a sad fact that most of us would like a magic wand to be waved and for things to be put right without any effort. Undergoing counselling seems rather frightening and you may fear, whether you admit it or not, that it could throw up some painful thoughts or memories. Overhauling your diet sounds far too bothersome and exercising regularly far too sweaty! It is hard to make the effort – we want it done for us with one easy pill. But if, as I have suggested, PMS may well be an expression of our hidden angers and frustrations at being devalued and put out of control of our own lives, making that effort and doing that work may be exactly what we need to get back into control. Perhaps the first step to doing something about your PMS is not to be told by some 'expert' the surefire cure to get you better, but for you yourself to decide which treatment you want to try.

TREAT THE SYNDROME OR TREAT THE SYMPTOM?

If we had an easy answer for what causes PMS it would stand to reason that we would be better off dealing with it at source rather than picking off individual symptoms and getting you pills for your headaches, pills for bloating or pills for breast tenderness. But, as you have seen, we don't have a clear idea of exactly why PMS happens so treating individual symptoms may sometimes seem to be the only option. However, you could approach PMS in a far wider context and consider the situation holistically. Rather than treating the symptoms or the syndrome, what you then do is treat yourself to a lifestyle overhaul. This approach involves looking at your diet, the way you exercise, your environment and your relationships.

You should start with the least invasive treatment first. If you have been suffering from PMS for some time and feel that you've tried eating sensibly or exercising and that nothing has worked, you may want to demand pretty drastic action from your GP from the beginning. And if your GP has had other PMS patients who have not responded to treatment, he or she may be in such despair at the situation that you may well be able to put pressure on them to obtain such a response. But it's not likely to be your best option. You would be better off taking a structured approach and working your way steadily, from a change of lifestyle and counselling, through nutritional supplements, before you go anywhere near prescription drugs or even surgery.

Because there is such a range of possible causes and an equal variety of treatments, you don't have to feel under pressure to try any of them, or that you are being obstructive or unreasonable if you turn any down. This is something that you may need to discuss at length with your doctor. You may feel unhappy at accepting certain treatments. The message is that you shouldn't turn anything down out of hand without discussing it. You may be refusing for all the wrong reasons, and once you've had your fears taken seriously and had a proper explanation you may feel more at ease. But equally, if you don't like the sound of it don't let anyone persuade you that you are refusing the one cure that could help. There are likely to be other methods that are just as effective that would be acceptable to you.

On your own, and then with a doctor and/or with other advisers, a gradual approach may take you through the following steps in this sort of order:

- a look at your lifestyle;
- changes in your eating patterns;
- vitamin and mineral supplements;
- painkillers such as ibuprofen or aspirin;
- Mefenamic acid;
- counselling;
- alternative therapies – acupuncture, homoeopathy etc.;
- hormones;
- diuretics;
- other prescription drugs;
- surgery.

But you should experiment with what feels acceptable to you. Always remember that any therapy, whether self-help, alternative or conventional, may need some time to work. Give everything, from exercise to hormone therapy, at least several menstrual cycles of proper use before judging whether or not it may be helping. You can't expect instant, overnight cures, however much you may desperately want them.

A FINAL WORD

PMS can be beaten. It may seem a confusing condition with no one, clear-cut explanation and no one, clear-cut solution. While there are women who will tell you that PMS has given them no end of problems and has been resistant to any cure, there are many who have fought the condition and won. The key seems to be in taking charge for yourself, rather than sitting back and expecting someone else to do the work for you, or believing those who insist there is only one cause and only one cure. You do need to keep an open mind. If acupuncture works for you, use it. If progesterone works for you, use it. If counselling works for you, use it. One, if not several, if not all of the treatments contained in this book *will* give you the ability to improve that time in your menstrual cycle that at the moment may seem intolerable. Keep trying, because you just need to find it!

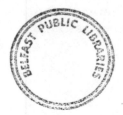

Useful Addresses

British Association for Counselling
1 Regent Place
Rugby
Warwicks CV21 2PJ
Tel: 01788 578328

British Herbal Medicine Association
1 Wickham Rd
Boscombe
Bournemouth BA7 6JX
Tel: 01202 433691

British Homoeopathic Association
27a Devonshire Street
London W1N 1RJ
Tel: 0171 935 2163

The British Wheel of Yoga
1 Hamilton Place
Boxton Road
Sleaford
Lincolnshire NG34 7ES
Tel: 01529 306851

Family Planning Association
27–35 Mortimer Street
London W1N 7RJ
Tel: 0171 636 7866

The FPA in Northern Ireland
113 University Street
Belfast BT7 1HP
Tel: 01232 325488

The FPA in Wales
Grace Phillips House
4 Museum Place
Cardiff CF1 3BG
Tel: 01222 342766

Health Education Authority
Hamilton House
Mabledon Place
London WC1H 9TX
Tel: 0171 383 3833

The Institute of Complementary Medicine
PO Box 194
London SE16 1QZ
Tel: 0171 237 5165

International Federation of Professional Aromatherapists
Hinckley and District Hospital
The Annexe
Mount Road
Hinckley
Leicestershire LE10 1AG

Marie Stopes House
108 Whitfield Street
London W1P 6BE
Tel: 0171 388 0662

National Association For Premenstrual Syndrome
PO Box 72
Sevenoaks
Kent TN13 1XQ
Tel: 01732 741709

National Childbirth Trust
Alexander House
Oldham Terrace
London W3 6NH
Tel: 0181 992 8637

The National Endometriosis Society
35 Belgrave Square
London SW1X 8OB
Tel: 0171 235 4137

PMS Help
PO Box 160
St Albans AL1 4YQ

Relate
Herbert Gray College
Little Church Street
Rugby CV21 3AP
Tel: 01788 73241

Women's Health Concern
PO Box 1629
London W8 6AU
Tel: 0171 938 3932

Women's Health and Reproductive Rights Information
Centre
52 Featherstone Street
London EC1Y 8RT
Tel: 0171 251 6580

The Women's Nutritional Advisory Service
PO Box 268
Lewes
East Sussex ·BN7 2QN
Tel: 01273 487366

Further Reading

Stress

The Good Stress Guide Mary Hartley (Sheldon Press)
Stress Leon Chaitow (Thorsons)
Understanding Stress Breakdown Dr William Wilkie (Millennium Books)

Self Esteem

Self Esteem Gael Lindenfield (Thorsons)

Counselling

The Counselling Handbook Susan Quilliam and Ian Grove-Stephensen (Thorsons)
Counselling and Psychotherapy Wendy Dryden and Colin Feltham (Sheldon Press)

Massage and Aromatherapy

The Magic Of Massage Ouida West (Century Publishing)
The Complete Book Of Massage Clare Maxwell-Hudson (Dorling Kindersley)

Super Massage Gordon Inkeles (Piatkus)
Aromatherapy – The Encyclopedia of Plants and Oils and How They Help You Daniele Ryman (Piatkus)
Aromatherapy Judith Jackson (Dorling Kindersley)

Yoga

Lyn Marshall's Yogacise Lyn Marshall (BBC Books)
Yogacise Vimla Lalvani (Hamlyn)

Natural Healing

Natural Healing for Women Susan Curtis and Romy Fraser (Pandora)
Herbal Medicine for Everyone Michael McIntyre (Penguin)
The A-Z of Nutritional Health Adrienne Mayes (Thorsons)
Encyclopaedia of Natural Medicine Michael Murray and Joseph Pizzorno (Optima)

Relaxation Tapes

Relaxation One to One Self Help Perry Lonsdale (Conifer Records)
Classic Relaxation Programme Dr Hilary Jones (Polygram)

References

Asso, D. & Magos, A. L. (1992) 'Psychological and physiological changes in severe premenstrual syndrome' *Biological Psychology 33.*

Bancroft, J. (1983) 'Mood, sexuality, hormones and the menstrual cycle. II. Hormone levels and their relationship to the premenstrual syndrome' *Psychosomatic Medicine 45.*

Bancroft, J. (1993) 'The premenstrual syndrome – a reappraisal of the concept and the evidence' *Psychological Medicine Supplement 24.*

Bancroft, J. & Backstrom, T. (1985) 'Premenstrual syndrome' *Clinical Endocrinology 22.*

Bancroft, J. & Rennie, D. (1993) 'The impact of oral contraceptives on the experience of perimenstrual mood, clumsiness, food craving and other symptoms' *Journal of Psychosomatic Research 37.*

Bancroft, J., Rennie, D. & Warner, P. (1993) 'Vulnerability to premenstrual mood change; the relevance of a past history of depressive disorder' *Psychosomatic Medicine (in the press).*

Bancroft, J. & Sartorius, N. (1990) 'The effects of oral contraceptives on wellbeing and sexuality' *Oxford Review of Reproductive Biology 22.*

Bancroft, J., Williamson, L., Warner, P., Rennie, D. & Smith, S. (1993) 'Perimenstrual complaints in women complaining of

PMS, menorrhagia and dysmenorrhoea: towards a dismantling of the premenstrual syndrome' *Psychosomatic Medicine 55.*

Bowen, D. J. & Grunberg, N. E. (1990) 'Variations in food preference and consumption across the menstrual cycle' *Physiology and Behavior 47.*

Dalton, K. (1984) *Premenstrual Syndrome and Progesterone Therapy* (Heinemann: London)

Dalton, K. & Holton, W. M. (1992) 'Diet of women with severe premenstrual syndrome and the effect of changing to a three-hourly starch diet' *Stress Medicine 8.*

Dennerstein, L., Spencer-Gardner, C., Gotts, G., Brown, J. B., Smith, M. A. and Burrows, G. D. (1985) 'Progesterone and the premenstrual syndrome: a double blind crossover trial' *British Medical Journal 290.*

Endicott, J., Halbreich, U., Schacht, S. & Nee, J. (1985) 'Affective disorder and premenstrual depression' In *Premenstrual Syndrome: Current Findings and Future Directions* (American Psychiatric Press: Washington DC)

Fradkin, B. & Firestone, P. (1986) 'Premenstrual tension, expectancy, and mother-child relations' *Journal of Behavioral Medicine 9.*

Greene, R. & Dalton, K. (1953) 'The premenstrual syndrome' *British Medical Journal 1.1007.*

Halbreich, U. & Endicott, J. (1982) 'Classification of premenstrual syndromes' In *Behaviour and the Menstrual Cycle* (Marcel Dekker, Inc.: New York)

Hammarback, S., Backstrom, T. & MacGibbon-Taylor, B. (1989) 'Diagnosis of premenstrual tension syndrome: description and evaluation of a procedure for diagnosis and differential diagnosis' *Journal of Psychosomatic Obstetrics and Gynaecology 10.*

Hargrove, J. T. & Abraham, G. E. (1982) 'The incidence of premenstrual tension in a gynaecologic clinic' *Journal of Reproductive Medicine 27.*

References

Haskett, R. F., Steiner, M., Osmun, J. N. & Carroll, B. J. (1980) 'Severe premenstrual tension: delineation of the syndrome' *Biological Psychiatry 15.*

Hurt, S. W., Schnurr, P. P., Severino, S. K., Freeman, E. W., Gise, L. H., Rivera-Tovar, A. & Steege, J. F. (1992) 'Late luteal phase dysphoric disorder in 670 women evaluated for premenstrual complaints' *American Journal of Psychiatry 149.*

Jakubowicz, D. L., Godard, E. & Dewhurst, J. (1984) 'The treatment of premenstrual tension with mefenamic acid: analysis of prostaglandin concentration' *British Journal of Obstetrics and Gynaecology 91.*

Kato, I. et al. (1989) 'Alcohol consumption in cancers of hormone related organs in females' *Japan Journal of Clinical Oncology 19, 3.*

Keye, W. R. Jr., Hammond, D. C. & Strang, T. (1986) 'Medical and psychological characteristics of women presenting with premenstrual symptoms' *Obstetrics and Gynaecology 68.*

Magos, A. L. & Studd, J. W. W. (1984) 'The premenstrual syndrome' In *Progress in Obstetrics and Gynaecology* (Churchill Livingstone: Edinburgh)

Mansel, R. E. (1988) 'Investigations and treatment of cyclical benign breast disease' In *Functional Disorders of the Menstrual Cycle* (Chichester: Wiley)

Moos, R. H. (1968) 'The development of menstrual distress questionnaire' *Psychosomatic Medicine 30.*

Morse, C. A. & Dennerstein, L. (1988) 'Cognitive therapy for premenstrual syndrome' In *Functional Disorders of the Menstrual Cycle* (Wiley: Chichester)

Muse, K. N., Cetel, N. S., Futterman, L. A. & Yen, S. S. C. (1984) 'The premenstrual syndrome. Effects of "medical ovariectomy" ' *New England Journal of Medicine 311.*

O'Keane, V., O'Hanlon, M., Webb, M. and Dinan, T. (1991) 'D-Fenfluramine/prolactin response throughout the menstrual cycle: evidence for an oestrogen-induced alteration' *Clinical Endocrinology 34.*

Olasov, B. & Jackson, J. (1987) 'Effects of expectancies on women's reports of moods during the menstrual cycle' *Psychosomatic Medicine 49*.

Parry, B. L. & Wehr, T. A. (1987) 'Theraputic effect of sleep deprivation in patients with premenstrual syndrome' *American Journal of Psychiatry 144*.

Plante, T. G. & Denney, D. R. (1984) 'Stress responsivity among dysmenorrheic women at different phases of their menstrual cycle: more ado about nothing' *Behaviour Research and Therapy 22*.

Reid, R. L. (1985) 'Premenstrual syndrome. Current Problems in Obstetrics' *Gynaecology and Fertility 8*.

Reid, R. L. (1986) 'Premenstrual syndrome: a time for introspection' *American Journal of Obstetrics and Gynaecology 155*.

Rosenburg, L. et al. (1982) 'Breast cancer and alcoholic beverage consumption' *Lancet 1*.

Rubinow, D. R. & Schmidt, P. J. (1992) 'Premenstrual syndrome: a review of endocrine studies' *Endocrinologist 2*.

Schmidt, P. J., Neiman, L., Grover, G. N., Muller, K. L., Merriam, G. R. & Rubinow, D. R. (1991) 'Lack of effect of induced menses on symptoms in women with premenstrual syndrome' *New England Journal of Medicine 324*.

Sommer, B. (1992) 'Cognitive performance and the menstrual cycle' In *Cognition and the Menstrual Cycle* (Springer-Verlag: New York)

Van den Akker, O. & Steptoe, A. (1985) 'The pattern and prevalence of symptoms during the menstrual cycle' *British Journal of Psychiatry 147*.

Van den Akker, O. & Steptoe, A. (1989) 'Psychophysiological responses in women reporting severe premenstrual symptoms' *Psychosomatic Medicine 51*.

Vergare, M. J. (1987) 'Premenstrual syndrome: implications for psychiatric practice' In *Premenstrual Syndrome: Ethical and Legal Implications in a Biomedical Perspective* (Plenum: New York)

References

Walker, A. & Bancroft, J. (1990) 'The relationship between premenstrual symptoms and oral contraceptive use: a controlled study' *Psychosomatic Medicine 52.*

Warner, P. & Bancroft, J. (1988) 'Mood, sexuality, oral contraceptives and the menstrual cycle' *Journal of Psychosomatic Research 32.*

Warner, P. & Bancroft, J. (1990) 'Factors related to the self-reporting of the premenstrual syndrome' *British Journal of Psychiatry 157.*

Warner, P., Bancroft, J., Dixson, A. & Hampson, M. (1991) 'The relationship between perimenstrual depressive mood and depressive illness' *Journal of Affective Disorders 23.*

Watson, N. R., Studd, J. W. W., Savvas, M., Garnett, T. & Baber, R. J. (1989) 'Treatment of severe premenstrual syndrome with oestroidal patches and cyclical oral norethisterone' *Lancet* ii, 730–732.

Watts, J. F., Butt, W. R. & Edwards, R. L. (1987) 'A clinical trial using danazol for the treatment of premenstrual tension' *British Journal of Obstetrics and Gynaecology 94.*

Watts, J. F., Butt, W. R., Edwards, R. L. & Holder, G. (1985) 'Hormonal studies in women with premenstrual tension' *British Journal of Obstetrics and Gynaecology 92.*

Wood, C. & Jakubowicz, D. (1980) 'The treatment of premenstrual symptoms with mefenamic acid' *British Journal of Obstetrics and Gynaecology 87.*

Woods, N. J., Most, A. & Deny, G. K. (1982) 'Prevalence of perimenopausal symptoms' *American Journal of Public Health 72.*

Zimmerman, E. & Parlee, M. B. (1973) 'Behavioral changes associated with the menstrual cycle: an experimental investigation' *Journal of Applied Psychology 3.*

Index

Piatkus Books

If you have enjoyed reading this book, you may be interested in other titles published by Piatkus.

Acupressure: How to Cure Common Ailments the Natural Way
Michael Reed Gach

The Alexander Technique   Liz Hodgkinson

Aromatherapy: The Encyclopedia of Plants and Oils and How They Help You   Daniele Ryman

Arthritis Relief at Your Fingertips: How to Use Acupressure Massage to Ease Your Aches and Pains   Michael Reed Gach

The Encyclopedia of Alternative Health Care   Kristin Olsen

Female Rage: How Women can Unlock their Rage and Empower their Lives   Mary Valentis & Anne Devane

Healing Breakthroughs: How Your Attitudes and Beliefs Can Affect Your Health   Dr Larry Dossey

Herbal Remedies: The Complete Guide to Natural Healing   Jill Nice

Infertility: Modern Treatments and the Issues they Raise   Maggie Jones

Losing Weight After Pregnancy   Elisabeth Bing and Libby Colman

Natural Remedies for Common Complaints   Belinda Grant Viagas

Super Massage   Gordon Inkeles

Women's Bodies, Women's Wisdom: The Complete Guide to Women's Health and Wellbeing   Dr Christine Northrup

Women's Cancers: The Treatment Options   Donna Dawson

For a free brochure with further information on our full range of titles, please write to:

Piatkus Books
Freepost 7 (WD 4505)
London W1E 4EZ

PIATKUS